Wound Care

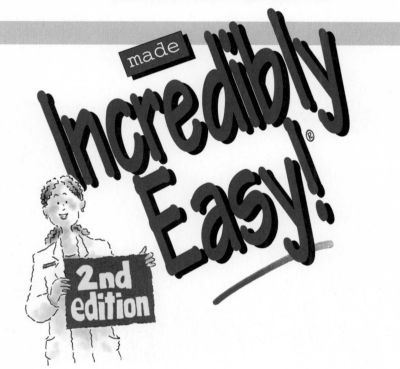

made **Incredibly Easy!**®

2nd edition

Wound Care

made **Incredibly Easy!**®

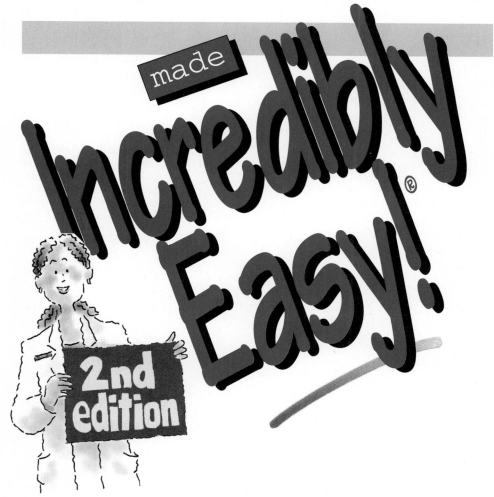

2nd edition

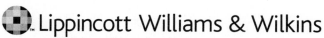

Lippincott Williams & Wilkins

a Wolters Kluwer business

Philadelphia · Baltimore · New York · London
Buenos Aires · Hong Kong · Sydney · Tokyo

Staff

Executive Publisher
Judith A. Schilling McCann, RN, MSN

Editorial Director
David Moreau

Clinical Director
Joan M. Robinson, RN, MSN

Art Director
Mary Ludwicki

Senior Managing Editor
Jaime Stockslager Buss, ELS

Editorial Project Manager
Coleen M.F. Stern

Clinical Project Manager
Beverly Ann Tscheschlog, RN, BS

Editor
Marcia A. Somerset

Clinical Editor
Pamela Kovach, RN, BSN

Copy Editors
Kimbery Bilotta (supervisor), Heather Ditch,
Danielle Michaely, Lisa Stockslager,
Dorothy P. Terry, Pamela Wingrod

Designer
Georg W. Purvis IV

Illustrator
Bot Roda

Digital Composition Services
Diane Paluba (manager), Joyce Rossi Biletz,
Donna S. Morris

Associate Manufacturing Manager
Beth J. Welsh

Editorial Assistants
Megan L. Aldinger, Karen J. Kirk, Linda K. Ruhf

Indexer
Karen C. Comerford

Library of Congress Cataloging-in-Publication Data
Wound care made incredibly easy.—2nd ed.
  p. ; cm.
  Includes bibliographical references and index.
  1. Wounds and injuries—Nursing. I. Lippincott Williams & Wilkins.
  [DNLM: 1. Wounds and Injuries—therapy—Handbooks. WO 39 W938 2007]
RD93.95.W68 2007
617.1'06—dc22
ISBN-13: 978-1-58255-539-3 (alk. paper)
ISBN-10: 1-58255-539-7 (alk. paper)   2006021598

Contents

Contributors and consultants

Monica A. Beshara, RN, BSN, CWOCN
Wound Care Specialist
DeKalb Medical Center
Decatur, Ga.

Phyllis A. Bonham, PhD, RN, MSN, CWOCN
Associate Professor and Director, Wound Care
  Education Program
College of Nursing
Medical University of South Carolina
Charleston, SC

Carol Calianno, RN, MSN, CWOCN
Wound, Ostomy, Continence Nurse Specialist
Jeanes Hospital — Temple Health System
Philadelphia

Margaret Davis, RN, MSN, PhD(c)
Assistant Professor of Nursing
Central Florida Community College
Ocala

Roxanne Leisky, MSN, MBA, FNP, CWS
Owner
Advanced Wound Care, LLC
Springfield, Ill.

Donna Scemons, RN, MSN, FNP-C, CWOCN, CNS
Family Nurse Practitioner
Healthcare Systems Inc.
Castaic, Calif.

Tracey J. Siegel, RN, MSN, CWOCN, NP
Instructor of Nursing
Charles E. Gregory School of Nursing
Perth Amboy, N.J.

Mary Sieggreen, APRN-BC, MSN, CVN
Nurse Practitioner Vascular Surgery
Harper University Hospital, Detroit Medical Center

Patricia Albano Slachta, APRN,BC, PhD, CWOCN
Clinical Nurse Specialist
Medical University of South Carolina
Charleston

Cynthia A. Worley, RN, BSN, COCN, CWCN
WOC Nurse
University of Texas M.D. Anderson Cancer Center
Houston

Karen Zulkowski, RN, DNS, CWS
Associate Professor
Montana State University
Bozeman

Foreword

Wound care is a dynamic, constantly changing field that has become increasingly outcome oriented with a focus on healing the wound, not just treating the etiology. Concern and interest regarding wound care has increased with an aging population and the expansion of patient care outside the acute care environment. Recognition that chronic and acute wound management greatly impacts the financial aspect of our health care system has propelled wound care into the limelight. This specialty has grown to encompass several health care professions, including nursing, medicine, physical therapy, and occupational therapy.

Wound Care Made Incredibly Easy, Second Edition, is an impressive reference for both the beginner and experienced practitioner. Theoretical as well as practical aspects of wound management are addressed within the text. A review of basic skin anatomy and physiology provides a foundation for understanding various etiologies of acute and chronic wounds. Chapters discussing treatment and dressing methodologies build on this knowledge and allow the practitioner to employ evidence-based wound care. Tried-and-true therapies are given equal billing with newer treatments. This edition also includes a new chapter on nonhealing wounds.

On top of that, it's fun! Illustrations, photographs, and charts present need-to-know concepts and procedures in an easy-to-understand and easy-to-read format. Two sections of color pages bring you a dramatic view of common wound types and complications as well as guide you through pressure ulcer staging. Appendices, such as the quick guide to wound care dressings and the wound and skin assessment tool, serve as tools you can use in your practice again and again. Quick quizzes at the end of each chapter test your knowledge and lighthearted characters throughout the book make learning fun and enjoyable.

Entertaining logos highlight key points:

Dress for success presents tips for choosing and applying wound dressings.

Get wise to wounds provides pointers for performing wound assessment, wound care procedures, and patient teaching.

Handle with care explains the unique wound care needs of pediatric, geriatric, and bariatric patients.

Memory joggers offer mnemonic devices and other learning aids to help reinforce difficult topics.

A quality wound management reference must address the needs of the wide variety of professionals in wound care. *Wound Care Made Incredibly Easy*, Second Edition, is a well-thought-out reference that provides sound information to benefit the expert and novice alike.

Kathryn Baxter, MS, FNP, CWOCN
Assistant Professor of Clinical Nursing
Colon & Rectal Surgery
Columbia University
New York

Wound care fundamentals

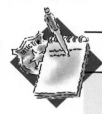

Just the facts

In this chapter, you'll learn:

♦ layers and functions of the skin

♦ types of wounds

♦ phases of wound healing

♦ factors that affect the skin's ability to heal

♦ complications of wound healing.

A look at the skin

The skin, or integumentary system, is the largest organ in the body. It accounts for about 6 to 8 lb (2.5 to 3.5 kg) of a person's body weight and has a surface area of more than 20 square feet. The thickest skin is located on the hands and on the soles of the feet; the thinnest skin, around the eyes and over the tympanic membranes in the ears.

Beauty's only skin deep

Skin protects the body by acting as a barrier between internal structures and the external world. Because skin also stands between each of us and the social world around us, we're also affected by its appearance. Healthy, unblemished skin with good tone (firmness) and color leads to a better self image. Skin also reflects the body's general physical health. For example, skin may look bluish if blood oxygen levels are low and it may appear flushed or red if a fever is present.

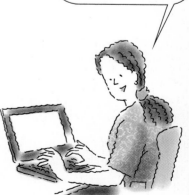

Wow! The skin makes up 6 to 8 lb of a person's weight. That's more than this laptop weighs!

A wound by any other name

Any damage to the skin is considered a wound. Wounds to the skin can result from planned events (such as surgery), accidents (such as a fall from a bike), or exposure to the environment (such as the damage caused by ultraviolet [UV] rays in sunlight).

Anatomy and physiology

Skin is composed of two main layers that function as a single unit: the epidermis and the dermis. The *epidermis* (outermost layer) is made up of five distinct layers. Covering the epidermis is the *keratinized epithelium*, a layer of cells that migrate up from the underlying dermis and die upon reaching the surface. These cells are continuously generated and replaced. The *dermis* (innermost layer) is made up of living cells that receive oxygen and nutrients through an extensive network of small blood vessels. In fact, every square inch of skin contains more than 15′ of blood vessels! A layer of subcutaneous fatty connective tissue, sometimes called the *hypodermis*, lies beneath these layers.

The skin you're in

Within the epidermis and dermis are five structural networks:
- collagen fibers
- elastic fibers
- small blood vessels
- nerve fibers
- lymphatic vessels.

These networks are stabilized by hair follicles and sweat gland ducts.

Epidermis

The epidermis — the outermost of the skin's two main layers — varies in thickness from about 0.1 mm thick on the eyelids to as much as 1 mm thick on the palms and soles. It's slightly acidic, with an average pH of 5.5.

In living color

The epidermis also contains melanocytes (cells that produce the brown pigment melanin), which give skin and hair their colors. The more melanin produced by melanocytes, the darker the skin. Skin color varies from one person to the next, but it can also vary from one area of the body to another. The hypothalamus regulates melanin production by secreting melanocyte-stimulating hormone.

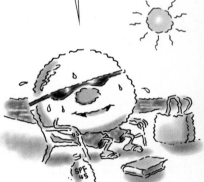

When my melanin kicks in, I'll be sporting a nice tan, but maybe I should start sporting some sunblock. These UV rays can be pretty damaging.

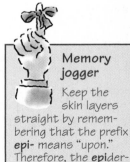

Memory jogger

Keep the skin layers straight by remembering that the prefix **epi-** means "upon." Therefore, the **epidermis** is upon, or on top of, the dermis.

The layered look

Each of the five layers of the epidermis has a name that reflects either its structure or its function. Let's look at them from the outside in:

• The *stratum corneum* (horny layer) is the superficial layer of dead skin cells (keratinized epithelium) that's in contact with the environment. This layer is separated by the dermis and underlying tissue. The stratum corneum has an acid mantle that helps protect the body from some fungi and bacteria. Cells in this layer continuously migrate through the stratum lucidum from the dermis below and die upon reaching the surface. These dead cells are shed daily and are completely replaced every 4 to 6 weeks. In diseases, such as eczema and psoriasis, the stratum corneum may become abnormally thick and irritate skin structures and peripheral nerves.

• The *stratum lucidum* (clear layer) is a single layer of cells that forms a transitional boundary between the stratum corneum above and stratum granulosum below. This layer is most evident in areas where skin is thickest such as on the soles. It appears to be absent in areas where skin is especially thin such as on the eyelids. Although cells in this layer lack active nuclei, this is an area of intense enzyme activity that prepares cells for the stratum corneum.

• The *stratum granulosum* (granular layer) is one to five cells thick and is characterized by flat cells with active nuclei. It's believed that this layer aids keratin formation.

• The *stratum spinosum* is the layer in which cells begin to flatten as they migrate toward the skin surface. Involucrin, a soluble protein precursor of the keratinized envelopes of skin cells, is synthesized here.

• The *stratum basale*, or *stratum germinativum*, is just one cell thick and is the only layer of the epidermis in which cells undergo mitosis to form new cells. The stratum basale forms the dermoepidermal junction—the area where the epidermis and dermis are connected. Protrusions of this layer (called *rete pegs* or *epidermal ridges*) extend down into the dermis where they're surrounded by vascularized dermal papillae. This unique structure supports the epidermis and facilitates the exchange of fluids and cells between the skin layers.

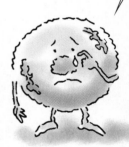

It's time for me to migrate to the skin's surface. I'll miss you stratum spinosum!

Dermis

The dermis—the thick, deeper layer of the skin—is composed of collagen and elastin fibers and an extracellular matrix, which contributes to the skin's strength and pliability. Collagen fibers give skin its strength, and elastin fibers provide elasticity. The meshing of collagen and elastin determines the skin's physical characteristics. (See *Structural supports: Collagen and elastin.*)

In addition, the dermis contains:
- blood vessels and lymphatic vessels, which transport oxygen and nutrients to cells and remove waste products
- nerve fibers and hair follicles, which contribute to skin sensation, temperature regulation, and excretion and absorption through the skin
- fibroblast cells, which are important in the production of collagen and elastin.

It takes two

The dermis is composed of two layers of connective tissue:
- The *papillary dermis* (outermost layer) is composed of collagen and reticular fibers, which are important in healing wounds. Capillaries in the papillary dermis carry the nourishment needed for metabolic activity in this layer.

Structural supports: Collagen and elastin

After you pull on the skin, it normally returns to its original position. This is because of the actions of the connective tissues collagen and elastin—two key components of skin.

Understanding the components
Collagen and elastin work together to support the dermis and give skin its physical characteristics.

Collagen
Collagen fibers form tightly woven networks in the papillary layer of the dermis — thick bundles that run parallel to the skin's surface. These fibers are relatively inextensible and nonelastic; therefore, they give the dermis high tensile strength. In addition, collagen constitutes about 70% of the skin's dry weight and is its principal structural body protein.

Elastin
Elastin is made up of wavy fibers that intertwine with collagen in horizontal arrangements at the lower dermis and vertical arrangements at the epidermal margin. Elastin makes skin pliable and is the structural protein that enables extensibility in the dermis.

Seeing the effects of age
As a person ages, collagen and elastin fibers break down and the fine lines and wrinkles that are associated with aging develop. Extensive exposure to sunlight accelerates this breakdown process. Deep wrinkles are caused by changes in facial muscles. Over time, laughing, crying, smiling, and frowning cause facial muscles to thicken and eventually cause wrinkles in the overlying skin.

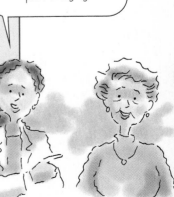

Don't let your laugh lines give you worry warts. Breakdown of collagen and elastin fibers is a normal part of aging.

• The *reticular dermis* (innermost layer) is formed by thick networks of collagen bundles that anchor it to the subcutaneous tissue and underlying supporting structures (such as fasciae, muscle, and bone).

Sebaceous glands and sweat glands

Although sebaceous glands and sweat glands appear to originate in the dermis, they're actually appendages of the epidermis that extend downward into the dermis.

Give these glands a hand!

Sebaceous glands, found primarily in the skin of the scalp, face, upper body, and genital region, are part of the same structure that contains hair follicles. These saclike glands produce sebum, a fatty substance that lubricates and softens the skin.

Don't sweat it

Sweat glands are tightly coiled and tubular; the average person has roughly 2.6 million of them. They're present throughout the body in varying amounts: the palms and soles have many but the external ear, lip margins, nail beds, and glans penis have none.

The secreting portion of the sweat gland originates in the dermis with its outlet on the surface of the skin. The sympathetic nervous system regulates sweat production, which, in turn, helps control body temperature.

Two types of sweat glands are present:

• *Eccrine* glands are active at birth and are found throughout the body. They're most dense on the palms, soles, and forehead. These glands connect to the skin's surface through pores and produce sweat that lacks proteins and fatty acids. Eccrine glands are smaller than apocrine glands.

• *Apocrine* glands begin to function at puberty. These glands open into hair follicles; therefore, most are found in areas where hair typically grows, such as the scalp, groin, and axillary region. The coiled secreting portion of each gland lies deep in the dermis (deeper than eccrine glands), and a duct connects it to the upper portion of the hair follicle. The sweat produced by apocrine glands contains water, sodium, chloride, proteins, and fatty acids. It's thicker than the sweat produced by eccrine glands and has a milky-white or yellowish tinge. (See *Oh no, B.O.!* page 6.)

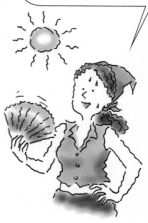

Along with this fan, my sympathetic nervous system helps keep me cool on hot days like this one. It really is "sympathetic," isn't it?

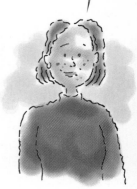

Apocrine sweat glands begin to function at puberty. Lucky me!

Oh no, B.O.!

The sweat produced by apocrine glands contains the same water, sodium, and chloride found in the sweat produced by eccrine glands; however, it also contains proteins and fatty acids. The unpleasant odor associated with sweat comes from the interaction of bacteria with these proteins and fatty acids.

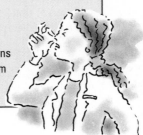

Subcutaneous tissue

Subcutaneous tissue, or hypodermis, is the subdermal (below the skin) layer of loose connective tissue that contains major blood vessels, lymph vessels, and nerves. Subcutaneous tissue:
• has a high proportion of fat cells and contains fewer small blood vessels than the dermis
• varies in thickness depending on body type and location
• constitutes 15% to 20% of a man's weight; 20% to 25% of a woman's weight
• insulates the body
• absorbs shocks to the skeletal system
• helps skin move easily over underlying structures.

Blood supply

The skin receives its blood supply through vessels that originate in underlying muscle tissue. Here, arteries branch into smaller vessels, which then branch into the network of capillaries that permeate the dermis and subcutaneous tissue.

Just passing through

Within the vascular system, only capillaries have walls thin enough (typically only a single layer of endothelial cells) to let solutes pass through. These thin walls allow nutrients and oxygen to pass from the bloodstream into the interstitial space around skin cells. At the same time, waste products pass into the capillaries and are carried away. The pressure of arterial blood entering the capillaries is about 30 mm Hg. The pressure of venous blood leaving the capillaries is about 10 mm Hg. This 20-mm Hg difference in pressure within the capillaries is quite low when compared with the pressure found in the larger arteries in the body (85 to 100 mm Hg), which is known as *blood pressure*. (See *Fluid movement through capillaries*.)

Fluid movement through capillaries

The movement of fluids through capillaries—a process called *capillary filtration*—results from blood pushing against the walls of the capillary. That pressure, called *hydrostatic* or *fluid-pushing pressure,* forces fluids and solutes through the capillary wall.

    When the hydrostatic pressure inside a capillary is greater than the pressure in the surrounding interstitial space, fluids and solutes inside the capillary are forced out into the interstitial space, as shown here. When the pressure inside the capillary is less than the pressure outside, fluids and solutes move back into it.

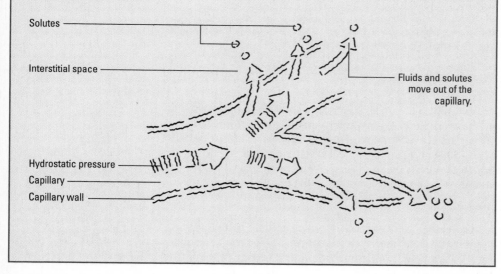

Solutes

Interstitial space

Fluids and solutes move out of the capillary.

Hydrostatic pressure

Capillary

Capillary wall

Lymphatic system

The skin's lymphatic system helps remove waste products, including excess proteins and fluids, from the dermis.

Go with the flow

Lymphatic vessels, or *lymphatics* for short, are similar to capillaries in that they're thin-walled, permeable vessels; however, lymphatics aren't part of the blood circulatory system. Instead, lymphatics belong to a separate system that removes proteins, large waste products, and excess fluids from the interstitial spaces in skin and then transports them to the venous circulation. The lymphatic vessels merge into two main trunks—the thoracic duct and the right lymphatic duct—which empty into the junction of the subclavian and internal jugular veins.

Functions of the skin

Skin performs, or participates in, a host of vital functions, including:
- protection of internal structures
- sensory perception
- thermoregulation
- excretion
- metabolism
- absorption
- social communication.

Damage to skin impairs its ability to carry out these important functions. Let's take a closer look at each.

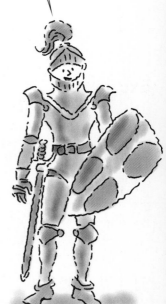

Sometimes you need more protection than at other times. Skin acts as a physical barrier to such invaders as microorganisms.

Protection

Skin acts as a physical barrier to microorganisms and foreign matter, protecting the body against infection by bacterial invasion. Two kinds of bacterial flora exist on the skin: *resident* (flora that lives on the skin) and *transient* (flora that isn't normally found on the skin). Most people carry at least five resident bacteria. Transient bacteria is removed by hand washing and bathing.

A thick skin

Skin also protects underlying tissue and structures from mechanical injury. Consider the feet: As a person walks or runs, the soles of the feet withstand a tremendous amount of force, yet the underlying tissue and bone structures remain unharmed.

Sensational stability

Finally, skin helps maintain a stable environment inside the body by preventing the loss of water, electrolytes, proteins, and other substances. Any damage jeopardizes this protection. When it's damaged, skin goes into repair mode to restore full protection by stepping up the normal process of cell replacement.

Sensory perception

Nerve endings in the skin allow a person to literally touch the world around him. Sensory nerve fibers originate in the nerve roots along the spine and supply specific areas of the skin known as *dermatomes*. Dermatomes are used to transmit sensory function. This same network helps a person avoid injury by making him aware of pain, pressure, heat, and cold.

Sensitivity training

Sensory nerves exist throughout the skin; however, some areas are more sensitive than others — for example, the fingertips are more sensitive than the back. Sensation allows us to identify potential dangers and avoid injury. Any loss or reduction of sensation (local or general) increases the chance of injury.

Sweat carries water to the skin's surface, at the same time preventing dehydration by making sure the body doesn't lose too much water.

Thermoregulation

Thermoregulation, or control of body temperature, involves the concerted effort of nerves, blood vessels, and eccrine glands in the dermis. When skin is exposed to cold or internal body temperature falls, blood vessels constrict, reducing blood flow and thereby conserving body heat.

Similarly, if skin becomes too hot or internal body temperature rises, small arteries within the skin dilate, increasing the blood flow, and sweat production increases to promote cooling.

Excretion

Although it may seem unlikely, the skin is an excretory organ. Excretion through the skin plays an important role in thermoregulation, electrolyte balance, and hydration. In addition, sebum excretion helps maintain the skin's integrity and suppleness.

Water works

Through its more than two million pores (small openings in the skin where sebum and sweat are released), the skin efficiently transmits trace amounts of water and body wastes to the environment. At the same time, it prevents dehydration by ensuring that the body doesn't lose too much water. Sweat carries water and salt to the skin surface, where it evaporates, aiding thermoregulation and electrolyte balance. In addition, a small amount of water evaporates directly from the skin itself each day. A normal adult loses about 500 ml of water a day this way. While the skin is busy regulating fluids that are leaving the body through sweat production, it's equally busy preventing unwanted or dangerous fluids from entering the body.

Metabolism

Skin also helps to maintain the mineralization of bones and teeth. A photochemical reaction in the skin produces vitamin D, which is crucial to the metabolism of calcium and phosphate. These minerals, in turn, play a central role in the health of bones and teeth. When skin is exposed to the UV spectrum in sunlight, vitamin D is synthesized in a photochemical reaction. Keep in mind, however, that overexposure to UV light causes damage that reduces the skin's ability to function properly.

Absorption

Some drugs and toxic substances (for example, pesticides) can be absorbed directly through the skin and into the bloodstream. This absorption process has been used to treat certain disorders via skin patch drug delivery systems. One example is the transdermal drug delivery method used in some nicotine withdrawal programs. This technology is also used to administer some forms of contraception, hormone replacement therapy, nitroglycerin, and some pain medications.

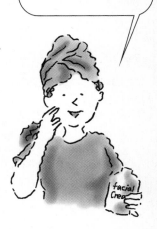

I'm not sure how I look right now, but I'm on my way to younger and healthier looking skin, according to the bottle. Watch out world!

Social communication

A commonly overlooked but important function of the skin is its role in self-esteem development and social communication. Every time a person looks in the mirror, he decides whether he likes what he sees. Although bone structure, body type, teeth, and hair all have an impact, the condition and characteristics of skin can have the greatest impact on a person's self-esteem. Ask any teenager with acne. If a person likes what he sees, self-esteem rises; if he doesn't, it sags.

You should have seen your face

Virtually every interpersonal exchange includes the nonverbal languages of facial expression and body posture. A person's level of self-esteem and skin characteristics — which are visible at all times — have an impact on how he communicates, both verbally and nonverbally, and how he's received by a listener.

Because the physical characteristics of skin are so closely linked to self-perception, a proliferation of skin care products and surgical techniques are available to keep skin looking young and healthy.

Aging and skin function

Over time, skin loses its ability to function as efficiently or as effectively as it once did. (See *How skin ages.*) As a result, advanced age places a person at greater risk for injuries, such as pressure ulcers and tumors, as well as various other skin conditions.

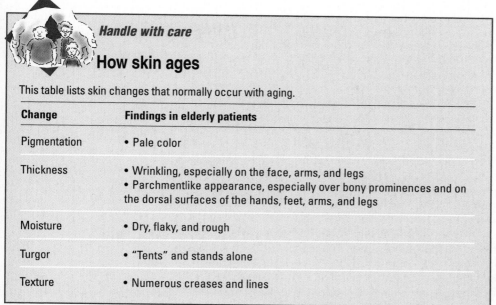

Handle with care

How skin ages

This table lists skin changes that normally occur with aging.

Change	Findings in elderly patients
Pigmentation	• Pale color
Thickness	• Wrinkling, especially on the face, arms, and legs • Parchmentlike appearance, especially over bony prominences and on the dorsal surfaces of the hands, feet, arms, and legs
Moisture	• Dry, flaky, and rough
Turgor	• "Tents" and stands alone
Texture	• Numerous creases and lines

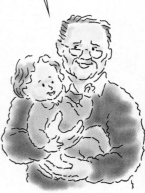

As a person ages, skin undergoes many changes that can increase the risk of wounds.

The road ahead

Although the entire body changes a great deal over time, several important changes in the skin increase the risk of wounds as a person ages. These include:
• a 50% reduction in the cell turnover rate in the stratum corneum (outermost layer) and a 20% reduction in dermal thickness
• generalized reduction in dermal vascularization and an associated drop in blood flow to the skin
• redistribution of subcutaneous tissue, which contains fewer fat cells in older people, to the stomach and thighs
• flattening of papillae in the dermoepidermal junction (meeting of the epidermis and dermis), which reduces adhesion between layers
• a drop in the number of Langerhans' cells (immune macrophages that attack invading germs) present in the skin
• a 50% decline in the number of fibroblasts and mast cells (cells that play a key role in the inflammatory response)
• marked reduction in the ability to sense pressure, heat, and cold, even though the same number of nerve endings in the skin are retained
• a significant decline in the number of sweat glands
• poorer absorption through the skin
• a reduction in the skin's ability to synthesize vitamin D.

Injury alert

As a person ages, physiologic changes also increase the risk of various injuries. For example, older adults:

• bruise easier and are more prone to edema around wounds due to reduced skin vascularization

• are more likely to suffer pressure and thermal (hot and cold) damage to the skin due to diminished sensation

• have a higher incidence of ischemia (cell damage resulting from too little oxygen reaching cells) in compressed tissue because bony areas have less subcutaneous cushioning and decreased sensation causes an elderly person to be less sensitive to the discomfort of remaining in one position for too long

• risk hyperthermia and hypothermia because of decreased subcutaneous tissue

• have fewer sweat glands and, therefore, produce less sweat, which hinders thermoregulation and increases the risk of hyperthermia

• have a higher risk of infection because thinner skin is a less effective barrier to germs and allergens and because the skin contains fewer Langerhans' cells to fight infection and fewer mast cells to mediate the inflammatory response

• are slower to exhibit a sensitization response (redness, heat, discomfort) due to the reduction in Langerhans' cells, resulting in overuse of topical medications and more severe allergic reactions (because signs aren't evident early on)

• risk overdose of transdermal medications when poor absorption prompts them to reapply the medication too often

• have a much higher incidence of shear and tear injuries due to compromised skin layer adhesion and less flexible collagen.

A look at wounds

Any break in the skin is considered a wound. Tissue damage in wounds varies widely, from a superficial break in the epithelium to deep trauma that involves the muscle and bone. A "clean" wound is a wound produced by surgery. A wound is described as "dirty" if it contains bacteria or other debris. Trauma typically produces dirty wounds. The rate of wound recovery varies according to the extent and type of damage incurred and other intrinsic factors, such as the patient's circulation, nutrition, and hydration. Although the recovery rate varies, the healing process is much the same in all cases.

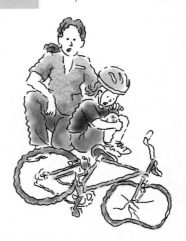

Trauma can cause some pretty dirty wounds.

Types of wound healing

A wound is classified by the way it closes. A wound can close by primary, secondary, or tertiary intention.

Primary intention

Primary intention involves reepithelialization, in which the skin's outer layer grows closed. Cells grow in from the margins of the wound and out from epithelial cells lining the hair follicles and sweat glands.

Just a scratch

Wounds that heal by primary intention are, most commonly, superficial wounds that involve only the epidermis with no loss of tissue—a first-degree burn, for example. A wound that has well-approximated edges (edges that can be pulled together to meet neatly), such as a surgical incision, also heals by primary intention. Because there's no loss of tissue and little risk of infection, the healing process is predictable. These wounds usually heal in 4 to 14 days and result in minimal scarring.

Secondary intention

Wounds that involve some degree of tissue loss with edges that can't be easily approximated heal by secondary intention. Depending on a wound's depth, it can be described as partial thickness or full thickness:
• Partial-thickness wounds extend through the epidermis and into, but not through, the dermis.
• Full-thickness wounds extend through the epidermis and dermis and may involve subcutaneous tissue, muscle and, possibly, bone.

Got you under my skin

During healing, wounds that heal by secondary intention fill with granulation tissue; then a scar forms and reepithelialization occurs, primarily from the wound edges. Pressure ulcers, burns, dehisced surgical wounds, and traumatic injuries are examples of this type of wound. These wounds also take longer to heal, result in scarring, and have a higher rate of complications than wounds that heal by primary intention.

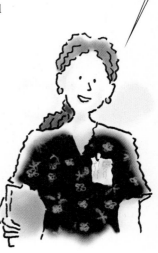

Wounds may heal by primary, secondary, or tertiary intention.

Tertiary intention

Wound that are intentionally kept open to allow edema or infection to resolve or to permit removal of exudate heal by tertiary intention (also called *delayed primary intention*). These wounds are later closed with sutures, staples, or adhesive skin closures. Wounds that heal by tertiary intention result in more scarring than wounds that heal by primary intention but less than wounds that heal by secondary intention.

Phases of wound healing

Whether the cause is mechanical, chemical, or thermal, the healing process is the same for all wounds. The wound healing process involves four specific phases:

* hemostasis
* inflammation
* proliferation
* maturation.

Although this categorization is useful, it's important to remember that healing rarely occurs in this strict order. Typically, the phases of wound healing overlap. (See *How wounds heal.*)

Hemostasis

Immediately after an injury, the body releases chemical mediators and intercellular messengers called *growth factors* that begin the process of cleaning and healing the wound.

Slow that flow!

When blood vessels are damaged, the small muscles in the walls of the vessels contract (vasoconstriction), reducing the flow of blood to the injury and minimizing blood loss. Vasoconstriction can last as long as 30 minutes, a process known as *hemostasis*.

Next, blood leaking from the inflamed, dilated, or broken vessels begins to coagulate. Collagen fibers in the wall of the damaged blood vessels activate the platelets in the blood that's in the wound. Aided by the action of prostaglandins, the platelets enlarge and stick together to form a temporary plug in the blood vessel, which helps prevent further bleeding. The platelets also release additional vasoconstrictors, such as serotonin, which help to prevent further blood loss. Thrombin forms in a cascade of events stimulated by the platelets, and a clot forms to close the small vessels and stop bleeding.

The initial phase of wound healing occurs almost immediately after the injury occurs and works quickly (within minutes) in small wounds. Hemostasis is less effective in stopping the bleeding in larger wounds.

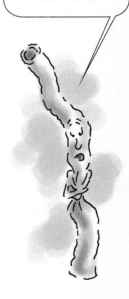

Vasoconstriction reduces the flow of blood to the injury, minimizing blood loss and promoting hemostasis.

How wounds heal

The healing process begins at the instant of injury and proceeds through a repair "cascade," as outlined here.

1. When tissue is damaged, serotonin, histamine, prostaglandins, and blood from the injured vessels fill the area. Blood platelets form a clot, and fibrin in the clot binds the wound edges together.

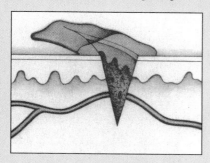

2. Lymphocytes initiate the inflammatory response, increasing capillary permeability. Wound edges swell; white blood cells from surrounding vessels move in and ingest bacteria and cellular debris, demolishing the clot. Redness, warmth, swelling, pain, and loss of function may occur.

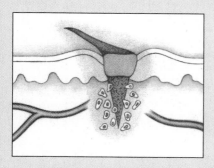

3. Adjacent healthy tissue supplies blood, nutrients, fibroblasts, proteins, and other building materials needed to form soft, pink, and highly vascular granulation tissue, which begins to bridge the area. Inflammation may decrease, or signs and symptoms of infection (increased swelling, increased pain, fever, and pus-filled discharge) may develop.

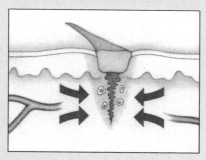

4. Fibroblasts in the granulation tissue secrete collagen, a gluelike substance. Collagen fibers crisscross the area, forming scar tissue.

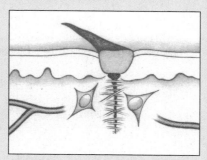

Meanwhile, epithelial cells at the wound edge multiply and migrate toward the wound center. A new layer of surface cells replaces the layer that was destroyed. New, healthy tissue or granulation tissue (if the blood supply is inadequate) appears.

5. Damaged tissue (including lymphatics, blood vessels, and stromal matrices) regenerates. Collagen fibers shorten, and the scar diminishes in size. Scar size may decrease and normal function may return or the scar may hypertrophy, leading to the formation of a keloid and the development of contractures.

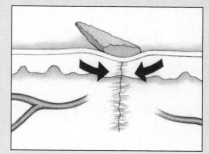

Inflammation

The inflammatory phase is both a defense mechanism and a crucial component of the healing process in which the wound is cleaned and rebuilding begins. (See *Understanding the inflammatory response.*)

During the inflammatory phase, vascular permeability increases, permitting serous fluid carrying small amounts of cell and plasma protein to accumulate in the tissue around the wound (edema). The accumulation of fluid causes the damaged tissue to appear swollen, red, and warm to the touch.

Search and destroy

During the early phase of the inflammatory process, neutrophils (one type of white blood cell) enter the wound. The primary role of neutrophils is phagocytosis (removal and destruction of bacteria and other contaminants).

As neutrophil infiltration slows, monocytes appear. Monocytes are converted into activated macrophages and continue the job of cleaning the wound. The macrophages play a key role early in the process of granulation and reepithelialization by producing growth factors and by attracting the cells needed for the formation of new blood vessels and collagen.

Telling time

The inflammatory phase of healing is important for preventing wound infection. The process is negatively influenced if the patient has a systemic condition that suppresses his immune system or if he's undergoing immunosuppressive ther-

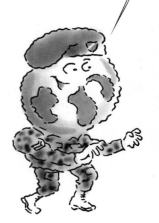

My mission's code name is phagocytosis. My orders are to infiltrate wounds and remove and destroy contaminants.

Understanding the inflammatory response

This flowchart outlines the sequence of events in the inflammatory process.

Microorganisms invade damaged tissue.

Basophils release heparin, and histamine and kinin production occurs.

Vasodilation occurs along with increased capillary permeability.

Blood flow increases to the affected tissues and fluid collects within them.

Neutrophils flock to the invasion site to engulf and destroy microorganisms from dying cells.

This sets the stage for the next phase: proliferation.

apy. In clean wounds, the inflammatory response lasts about 36 hours. In dirty or infected wounds, the response can last much longer.

Proliferation

During the proliferation phase of the healing process, the body:
• fills the wound with connective tissue (granulation)
• contracts the wound edges (contraction)
• covers the wound with epithelium (epithelialization).

Presto change-o!

All wounds go through the proliferation phase, but it takes much longer in wounds with extensive tissue loss. Although phases overlap, wound granulation generally starts when the inflammatory response is complete. As the inflammatory phase subsides, wound exudate (drainage) begins to decrease.

The proliferation phase involves regeneration of blood vessels (angiogenesis) and the formation of connective or granulation tissue. The development of granulation tissue requires an adequate supply of blood and nutrients. Endothelial cells in the blood vessels of the surrounding tissue reconstruct damaged or destroyed vessels by first migrating and then proliferating to form new capillary beds. As the beds form, this area of the wound takes on a red, "beefy," granular appearance. This tissue is a good defense against contaminants, but it's also quite fragile and bleeds easily.

Let the rebuilding begin

During the proliferation phase, growth factors prompt fibroblasts to migrate to the wound. Fibroblasts are the most common cell in connective tissue. They're responsible for making fibers and ground substance (also known as *extracellular matrix*), which provides support to cells. At first, fibroblasts populate just the margins of the wound; they later spread over the entire wound surface.

Fibroblasts have the important task of synthesizing collagen fibers which, in turn, produce keratinocyte, a growth factor needed for reepithelialization. This process necessitates a delicate balance of collagen synthesis and lysis (making new and removing old collagen). If the process yields too much collagen, increased scarring results. If the process yields too little collagen, scar tissue is weak and easily ruptured. Because fibroblasts require a supply of oxygen to perform their important role, capillary bed regeneration is crucial to the process.

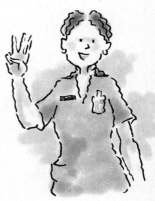

Granulation, contraction, and epithelialization are the three stages of the proliferation phase.

Pulling it all together

As healing progresses, myofibroblasts and the newly formed collagen fibers contract, pulling the wound edges toward each other. Contraction reduces the amount of granulation tissue needed to fill the wound, which speeds the healing process. (See *Contraction vs. contracture.*)

Complete healing occurs only after epithelial cells have completely covered the surface of the wound. When this occurs, keratinocytes switch from a migratory mode to a differentiation mode. The epidermis thickens and becomes differentiated, and the wound is closed. Any remaining scab comes off and the new epidermis is toughened by the production of keratin, which also returns the skin to its original color.

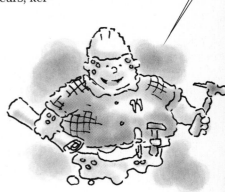

Fibroblasts may be small but we have a big job. We synthesize collagen, which is necessary for proper wound healing.

Maturation

The final phase of wound healing is maturation, which is marked by the shrinking and strengthening of the scar. This is a gradual, transitional phase of healing that can continue for months or even years after the wound has closed.

Movin' on

During maturation, fibroblasts leave the site of the wound, vascularization is reduced, the scar shrinks and becomes pale, and the mature scar forms. If the wound involved extensive tissue destruction, the scar won't contain hair, sweat, or sebaceous glands.

The wound gradually gains tensile strength. In wounds that heal by primary intention, tissues will achieve about 30% to 50% of

---

Contraction vs. contracture

Contraction and contracture occur during the wound healing process. While they have mechanisms in common, it's important to understand how contraction and contracture differ:

• Contraction, a desirable process that occurs during healing, is the process by which the edges of a wound pull toward the center of the wound to close it. Contraction continues to close the wound until tension in the surrounding skin causes it to slow and then stop.

• Contracture is an undesirable process and a common complication of burn scarring. Typically, contracture occurs after healing is complete. Contracture involves an inordinate amount of pulling or shortening of tissue, resulting in an area of tissue with only limited ability to move. It's especially problematic over joints, which may be pulled to a flexed position. Stretching is the only way to overcome contracture, and patients typically require physical therapy.

their original strength between days 1 and 14. When fully healed, tissue will achieve, at best, about 80% of its original strength. Scar tissue will always be less elastic than the surrounding skin.

Factors that affect healing

The healing process is affected by many factors. The most important influences include:
- nutrition
- oxygenation
- infection
- age
- chronic health conditions
- medications
- smoking.

Nutrition

Proper nutrition is arguably the most important factor in wound healing; however, malnutrition is a common finding among patients with wounds. It's reported in 30% of adult surgical patients and 45% to 57% of nonsurgical patients. For older adults, the problem is more pervasive. Malnutrition is reported in 53% to 74% of older hospitalized patients.

Poor nutrition prolongs hospitalization and increases the risk of medical complications. The severity of complications is directly related to the severity of the malnutrition. In older patients, malnutrition is known to increase the risk of pressure ulcers and delay wound healing. It may also contribute to poor tensile strength in healing wounds, with an associated increase in the risk of wound dehiscence. (See *Tips for detecting nutritional problems*, page 20.)

Protein power

Protein is crucial for wounds to heal properly. In fact, a person needs to double the recommended dietary allowance of protein (from 0.8 to 1.6 g/kg/day) before tissue even begins to heal. If a significant amount of body weight has been lost in connection with the injury, as much as 50% of the lost weight must be regained before healing will begin. A patient who lacks protein reserves heals slowly, if at all, and a patient who's borderline malnourished can easily become malnourished under this demand.

The body needs protein to form collagen during the proliferation phase. Without adequate protein, collagen formation is reduced or delayed and the healing process slows. Studies of malnourished patients indicate that they have lower levels of serum

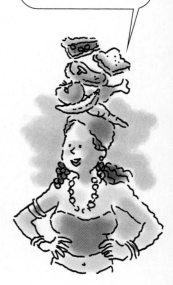

Because nutrition plays a critical role in wound healing, you need to make sure that your patient eats a balanced diet.

Tips for detecting nutritional problems

Nutritional problems may stem from physical conditions, drugs, diet, or lifestyle factors. The list below can help you identify risk factors that make your patient particularly susceptible to nutritional problems.

Physical condition
- Chronic illnesses (such as diabetes) and neurologic, cardiac, or thyroid problems
- Family history of diabetes or heart disease
- Draining wounds or fistulas
- Weight issues—weight loss of 5% of normal body weight; weight less than 90% of ideal body weight; weight gain or loss of 10 lb (4.5 kg) or more in last 6 months; obesity; or weight gain of 20% above normal body weight
- History of GI disturbances
- Anorexia or bulimia
- Depression or anxiety
- Severe trauma
- Recent chemotherapy or radiation therapy
- Physical limitations, such as paresis or paralysis

- Recent major surgery
- Pregnancy, especially teen or multiple-birth pregnancy

Drugs and diet
- Fad diets
- Steroid, diuretic, or antacid use
- Mouth, tooth, or denture problems
- Excessive alcohol intake
- Strict vegetarian diet
- Liquid diet or nothing by mouth for more than 3 days

Lifestyle factors
- Lack of support from family or friends
- Financial problems

albumin, which results in slower oxygen diffusion and, in turn, a reduction in the ability of neutrophils to kill bacteria. Wound exudate alone can contain up to 100 g of protein per day.

Nifty nutrients

Fatty acids (lipids) are used in cell structures and play a role in the inflammatory process. Also, vitamins C, B-complex, A, and E and the minerals iron, copper, zinc, and calcium are important in the healing process. A zinc deficiency adversely affects the proliferation phase by slowing the rate of epithelialization and decreasing the strength of collagen produced—and, thus, the strength of the healing skin.

In addition to protein and zinc, collagen synthesis requires supplies of carbohydrates and fat. Collagen cross-linking requires adequate amounts of vitamins A and C, iron, and copper. Vitamin C, iron, and zinc are important to developing tensile strength during the maturation phase of wound healing.

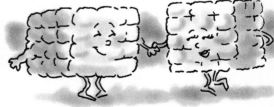

Protein is a critical component of wound healing. Double up on your patient's protein intake to ensure proper and timely healing.

Oxygenation

Wound healing depends on a regular supply of oxygen. For example, oxygen is critical for leukocytes to destroy bacteria and for fibroblasts to stimulate collagen synthesis. If the supply is hindered by poor blood flow to the area of the wound or if the patient's ability to take in adequate oxygen is impaired, the result is the same — impaired healing.

Possible causes of inadequate blood flow to the area of the wound include pressure, arterial occlusion, or prolonged vasoconstriction, possibly associated with such medical conditions as peripheral vascular disease and atherosclerosis. Possible causes of a lower than necessary systemic blood oxygenation include:
- inadequate oxygen intake
- hypothermia or hyperthermia
- anemia
- alkalemia
- other medical conditions such as chronic obstructive pulmonary disease.

Infection

Infection can be systemic or localized in the wound. A systemic infection, such as pneumonia or tuberculosis, increases the patient's metabolism and thus consumes the fluids, nutrients, and oxygen that the body needs for healing.

Damaging developments

A localized infection in the wound itself is more common. Remember, any break in the skin allows bacteria to enter. The infection may occur as part of the injury or may develop later in the healing process. For example, when the inflammatory phase lingers, wound healing is delayed and metabolic by-products of bacterial ingestion accumulate in the wound. This buildup interferes with the formation of new blood vessels and the synthesis of collagen. Infection can also occur in a wound that has been healing normally. This is especially true for larger wounds involving extensive tissue damage. New or increased pain, redness, heat, and drainage are signs of a new infection. In any case, healing can't progress until the cause of infection is addressed.

Age

Skin changes that occur with aging can prolong healing time in elderly patients. Although delayed healing is partially due to physiologic changes, it's usually complicated by other problems associated with aging, such as poor nutrition and hydration, the presence

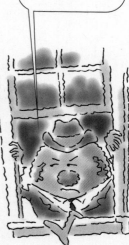

Pay no attention to me! I'm just looking for a way to get under your skin.

of a chronic condition, or the use of multiple medications. (See *Effects of aging on wound healing.*)

Chronic health conditions

Respiratory problems, atherosclerosis, diabetes, and malignancies can increase the risk of wounds and interfere with wound healing. These conditions can interfere with systemic and peripheral oxygenation and nutrition, which affect healing.

Getting complicated

Impaired circulation, a common problem for patients with diabetes and other disorders, can cause tissue hypoxia (lack of oxygen). Neuropathy associated with diabetes reduces a person's ability to sense pressure. As a result, a diabetic patient may experience trauma, especially to the feet, without realizing it. Insulin dependency can impair leukocyte function, which adversely affects cell proliferation.

Hemiplegia and quadriplegia involve the breakdown of muscle tissue and reduction in the padding around the large bones of the lower body. Because a patient with one of these conditions lacks sensation, he's at risk for developing chronic pressure ulcers.

Other conditions that can delay healing include dehydration, end-stage renal disease, thyroid disease, heart failure, peripheral vascular disease, and vasculitis and other collagen vascular disorders.

(Text continues on page 23.)

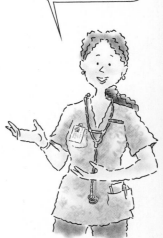

Don't forget that such health problems as respiratory disorders, atherosclerosis, diabetes, and malignancies not only increase the risk of wounds but also hinder healing.

Handle with care

Effects of aging on wound healing

In older adults, the following factors impede wound healing:
- slower turnover rate in epidermal cells
- poorer oxygenation at the wound due to increasingly fragile capillaries and a reduction in skin vascularization
- altered nutrition and fluid intake resulting from physical changes that can accompany aging, such as reduced saliva production, a declining sense of smell and taste, or decreased stomach motility
- altered nutrition and fluid intake attributable to troubling personal or social issues, such as loose-fitting dentures, financial concerns, eating alone after the death of a spouse, or problems preparing or obtaining food
- impaired function of the respiratory or immune systems
- reduced dermal and subcutaneous mass leading to an increased risk of chronic pressure ulcers
- healed wounds that lack tensile strength and are prone to reinjury.

A close look at skin layers

Skin is made up of separate layers that function as a single unit. Two distinct layers of skin, the epidermis and dermis, lie above a layer of subcutaneous fatty tissue (sometimes called the *hypodermis*).

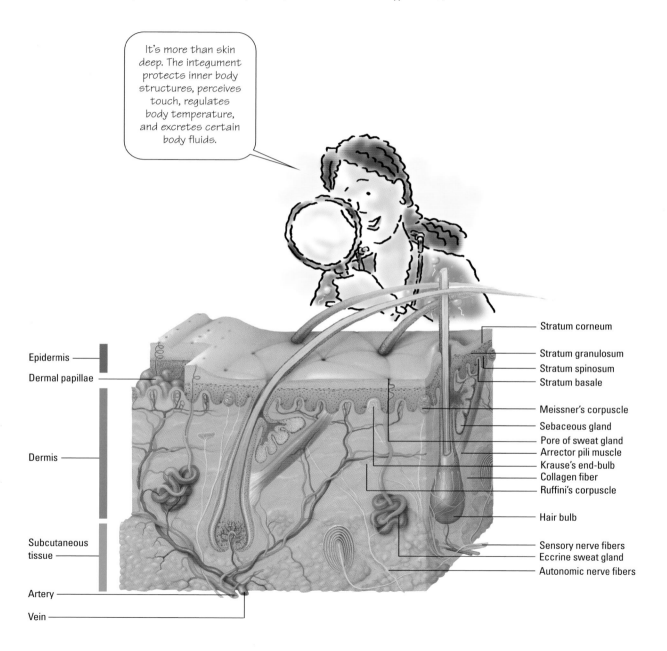

It's more than skin deep. The integument protects inner body structures, perceives touch, regulates body temperature, and excretes certain body fluids.

Epidermis

Dermal papillae

Dermis

Subcutaneous tissue

Artery

Vein

Stratum corneum

Stratum granulosum

Stratum spinosum

Stratum basale

Meissner's corpuscle

Sebaceous gland

Pore of sweat gland

Arrector pili muscle

Krause's end-bulb

Collagen fiber

Ruffini's corpuscle

Hair bulb

Sensory nerve fibers

Eccrine sweat gland

Autonomic nerve fibers

Wound bed condition

Wound bed appearance can guide your specific management approach and tell you how well a wound is healing.

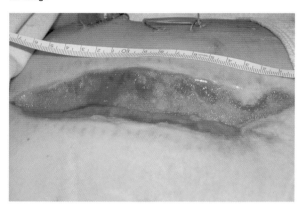

Granulation tissue

When a wound begins to heal, a layer of pale pink granulation tissue covers the wound bed. As this layer thickens, it becomes beefy red. This photo shows a granulation tissue base in an abdominal wound.

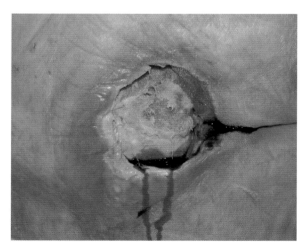

Fibrin slough

Yellow slough or dead tissue on the wound base is usually fibrin left over from the healing process. This slough, or soft necrotic tissue, is a medium for bacteria growth. This photo shows a sacral pressure ulcer with three quarters of the surface area covered with yellow necrotic slough.

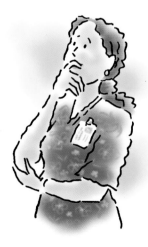

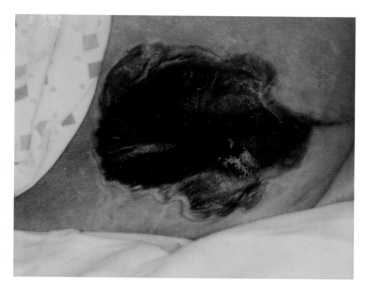

Eschar

Eschar signals necrosis. Dead avascular tissue slows healing and provides a site for microorganisms to proliferate. The photo at left shows a pressure ulcer with eschar; the photo below shows black ischemic toe ulcers.

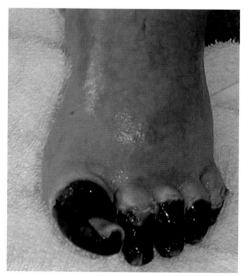

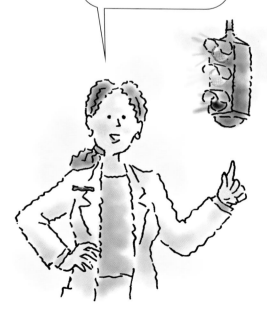

Detecting wound dehiscence

Although surgical wounds typically heal without incident, occasionally the edges of a wound may fail to join or may separate after they begin to heal. This development, called *wound dehiscence,* may lead to evisceration, an even more serious complication in which a portion of a viscus (in an abdominal incision, usually a bowel loop) protrudes through the incision. These photos illustrate a dehisced abdominal wound and a dehisced, healing abdominal incision.

Dehisced abdominal wound (with a colostomy)

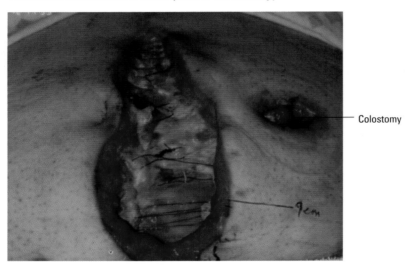

Colostomy

Dehisced, healing abdominal incision

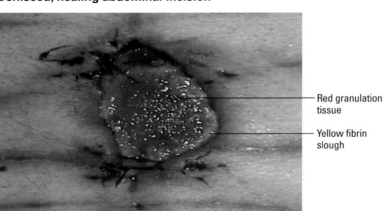

Red granulation tissue

Yellow fibrin slough

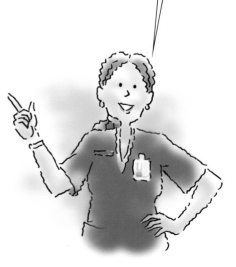

Note the red granulation tissue in the center and the yellow fibrin slough at the wound bed edges.

Day and night shifts

Normally, a healthy person shifts position every 15 minutes or so, even during sleep. This prevents tissue damage due to ischemia. Anything that impairs the ability to sense pressure, including the use of pain medications, spinal cord lesions, or cognitive impairment, puts the patient at risk for trauma (the patient can't feel the growing discomfort of pressure and respond to it).

Medications

Any medications that reduce a patient's movement, circulation, or metabolic function, such as sedatives and tranquilizers, have the potential to inhibit his ability to sense and respond to pressure. Also, because movement promotes adequate oxygenation, lack of motion means that peripheral blood delivers less oxygen to the extremities than it should. This is especially problematic for older adults. Remember, oxygen is important; without it, the healing process slows and the potential for complications rises.

At a turtle's pace

Some medications, such as steroids and chemotherapeutic agents, reduce the body's ability to mount an appropriate inflammatory response. This interrupts the inflammatory phase of healing and can dramatically lengthen healing time, especially in patients with compromised immune systems.

Smoking

Carbon monoxide, a component of cigarette smoke, binds to the hemoglobin in blood in the place of oxygen. This significantly reduces the amount of oxygen circulating in the bloodstream, which can impede wound healing. To some extent, this reaction also occurs in people regularly exposed to second-hand smoke.

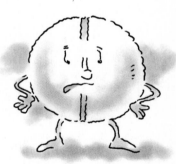

Medications, particularly sedatives, can also cause wound healing complications.

Complications of wound healing

The most common complications associated with wound healing are hemorrhage, dehiscence and evisceration, and infection.

Hemorrhage

Internal hemorrhage (bleeding) can result in the formation of a hematoma—a blood clot that solidifies to form a hard lump under the skin. Hematomas are commonly found around bruises.

External hemorrhage is visible bleeding from the wound. External bleeding during healing isn't unusual because the newly developed blood vessels are fragile and rupture easily. This is one reason that a wound needs to be protected by a dressing. However, each time the new blood vessels suffer damage, healing is delayed while repairs are made.

Dehiscence and evisceration

Dehiscence is a separation of the skin and underlying tissue layers. It's most likely to occur 3 to 11 days after the injury is sustained and may follow surgery. Evisceration is similar but involves the protrusion of underlying visceral organs as well. (See *Recognizing dehiscence and evisceration.*)

Dehiscence and evisceration may constitute a surgical emergency, especially if they involve an abdominal wound. If a wound opens without evisceration, it may need to heal by secondary intention. Poor nutrition and advanced age are two factors that increase a patient's risk of dehiscence and evisceration. Obesity also increases the risk of these complications. (See *Wound healing and the bariatric patient.*)

Infection

Infection is a relatively common complication of wound healing that should be addressed promptly. Infection can lead to a cellulitis or a bacterial infection that spreads to surrounding tissue. Signs of infection include:
• redness and warmth of the margins and tissue around the wound
• fever

Recognizing dehiscence and evisceration

In wound dehiscence, the layers of a wound separate. In evisceration, the viscera (in this case, a bowel loop) protrude through the wound.

Wound dehiscence

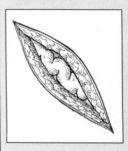

Evisceration of bowel loop

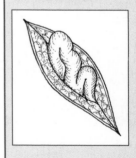

Handle with care

Wound healing and the bariatric patient

The bariatric patient is at risk for delayed wound healing due to:
• reduced tissue perfusion in adipose tissue and increased tension at the suture line caused by the weight of excess body fat
• excess skin folds (especially if the wound is within one of the folds or if the folds of excess tissue cover a suture line, which may keep the wound moist and allow bacteria to accumulate)
• associated medical conditions such as type 2 diabetes mellitus.

The bariatric patient is also at increased risk for dehiscence and evisceration because his diet may be seriously lacking in the essential minerals and vitamins that are necessary for proper wound healing.

- edema
- pain (or a sudden increase in pain)
- pus
- increase in exudate or a change in its color
- odor
- discoloration of granulation tissue
- further wound breakdown or lack of progress toward healing.

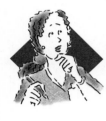

Quick quiz

1. The outermost layer of the skin is the:
    A. epidermis.
    B. dermis.
    C. hypodermis.
    D. subdermal layer.

Answer: A. The epidermis is the outermost layer of the skin. It's composed of epithelial tissue and is supported by the dermis.

2. The layer of skin that contains apocrine sweat glands is the:
    A. stratum corneum.
    B. dermis.
    C. subcutaneous tissue.
    D. stratum basale.

Answer: B. Apocrine glands are situated in the dermis and have ducts that empty into hair follicles.

3. The structures that deliver oxygen and nutrients to skin cells are:
    A. dermatomes.
    B. lymphatics.
    C. capillaries.
    D. quadratics.

Answer: C. A rich network of capillaries delivers oxygen to the skin's cells.

4. The main functions of the skin include:
    A. support, nourishment, and sensation.
    B. protection, sensory perception, and temperature regulation.
    C. fluid transport, sensory perception, and aging regulation.
    D. support, protection, and communication.

Answer: B. The skin's main functions involve protection from injury, noxious chemicals, and bacterial invasion; sensory perception of touch, temperature, and pain; and regulation of body heat.

5.   Which type of wound closes by primary intention?
  A.   Second-degree burn
  B.   Pressure ulcer
  C.   Traumatic injury
  D.   Surgical incision

Answer: D. A surgical incision is an example of a wound that closes by primary intention, in which there's no deep tissue loss and the wound edges are well approximated.

6.   Which phase of the wound healing process is responsible for cleaning the wound and starting the rebuilding process?
  A.   Hemostasis
  B.   Inflammation
  C.   Proliferation
  D.   Maturation

Answer: B. The inflammatory phase is both a defense mechanism that's vital to preventing infection of the wound and a crucial component of the healing process.

Scoring

☆☆☆   If you answered all six questions correctly, congrats! It looks like the information in this chapter has gotten under your skin.

☆☆   If you answered four or five questions correctly, good job! It's our sensory perception that you're well healed.

☆   If you answered fewer than four questions correctly, don't sweat it! After a quick review, this topic won't "phase" you at all.

Wound assessment and monitoring

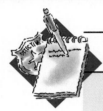

Just the facts

In this chapter, you'll learn:

♦ assessment methods

♦ ways to classify wounds according to type, age, and depth

♦ accurate documentation of wound progress

♦ tools to track wound healing.

Wound assessment

Each time you assess a wound, remember that you're assessing a patient with a wound — not simply the wound itself. This will help keep you focused on the big picture as you perform your initial assessment and will set the stage for effective monitoring and successful healing.

When you gather information about a wound, you must use all your senses. Be sure to cover the key assessment considerations below as well as assessing the wound bed and drainage. As you perform your assessment, remember that it doesn't matter what method you use to record your observations as long as you're consistent.

Key assessment considerations

Several factors influence the body's ability to heal itself, regardless of the type of injury suffered. You should include these elements in your wound assessment:
• immune status
• blood glucose levels, especially glycosylated hemoglobin (HbA_{1c})
• hydration
• nutrition
• blood albumin and pre-albumin levels

- oxygen and vascular supply
- pain
- cause of the wound.

Immune status

The immune system plays a central role in wound healing. If the patient's immune system is impaired due to diseases, such as human immunodeficiency virus infection, or as a result of chemotherapy or radiation, you should monitor the wound for impaired healing. Remember, chemotherapeutic agents aren't only used to treat cancer patients; they may also be used to treat inflammatory diseases such as arthritis. Corticosteroids may also depress immune system function.

Blood glucose levels

Blood glucose levels should be below 200 mg/dl for satisfactory healing, regardless of the wound's cause. Levels of 200 mg/dl or more can impair the function of white blood cells (WBCs), which are important in wound healing because they help prevent infection.

HbA_{1c} is also an indication of glucose control and the efficacy of diabetic therapy. An elevated HbA_{1c} level has the same consequences as an elevated blood glucose level: impaired wound healing and reduced ability to fight infection.

Hydration

Be sure to closely monitor and optimize the patient's hydration status — successful healing depends on it. Skin and subcutaneous tissues need to be well hydrated from the inside. Dehydration impairs the healing process by slowing the body's metabolism. Dehydration also reduces skin turgor, or fullness, leaving skin vulnerable to new wounds.

Nutrition

Nutritional status helps you determine the patient's vulnerability to skin breakdown as well as the body's overall ability to heal. A comprehensive assessment of the patient's nutritional status also helps you plan effective care. (See *Parts of a nutritional assessment.*)

Keep in mind that nutrition is complex. If your assessment leads you to believe that the patient's nutritional status places him at risk for skin damage or for delayed wound healing, collaborate with a dietitian to develop the best possible treatment plan.

Parts of a nutritional assessment

A comprehensive nutritional assessment can play an important part in wound care. Remember the four parts of a nutritional assessment, shown here.

HEALTH HISTORY

LABORATORY TESTS

BODY SYSTEMS ASSESSMENT

ANTHROPOMETRIC MEASUREMENTS

Blood albumin and pre-albumin levels

Blood albumin and pre-albumin levels are essential factors in wound assessment for two important reasons:

Skin is primarily constructed of protein, and albumin is a protein. If albumin levels are low, the body lacks an important building block for skin repair.

Albumin is the blood component that provides colloid osmotic pressure — the force that prevents fluid from leaking out of blood vessels into nearby tissues. (See *A closer look at albumin.*) If albumin levels fall below 3.5 g/dl, the patient can develop edema (fluid leakage into tissues), which compromises wound healing. The patient also risks developing hypotension (low blood pressure) as fluid leaks out of the bloodstream into tissues. If blood pressure falls to the point where adequate blood flow is no longer maintained through the capillaries near the wound, healing slows or stops.

A patient's pre-albumin level is a better indication of his nutritional status because a normal level (16 to 35 mg/dl) is less affected by liver and renal disease and hydration status than other serum proteins.

A closer look at albumin

Albumin, a large protein molecule, acts like a magnet to attract water and hold it inside the blood vessel.

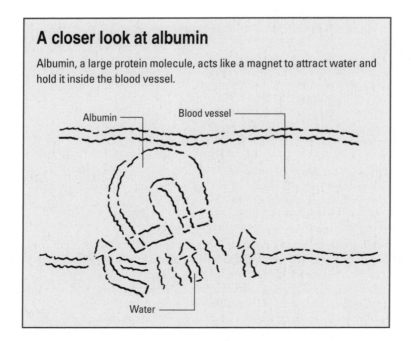

Oxygen and vascular supply

Healing requires oxygen — it's that simple. Therefore, anything that impedes full oxygenation also impedes healing. During your assessment, you should consider any factor that may reduce the amount of oxygen available for healing. Possible problems include:
- impaired gas exchange, causing decreased oxygen levels in the blood
- hemoglobin levels too low to transport adequate oxygen
- low blood pressure that fails to drive oxygenated blood through capillaries
- insufficient arterial and capillary supply in the wound area.

Any of these problems on their own or in combination can deprive the wound of the oxygen needed for successful healing.

Smoke bomb

Smoking is a modifiable factor that impedes oxygenation of the wound. If the patient is a smoker, explain to him ways in which smoking affects wound healing:
- Nicotine is a powerful vasoconstrictor that narrows peripheral blood vessels, thereby compromising blood flow to the skin.
- Because it's easier for hemoglobin to bind to the carbon monoxide present in cigarette smoke than it is for it to bind to oxygen, the blood that does squeeze through carries far less oxygen than it should.
- Lung tissue damaged by smoke doesn't function as well as it should, resulting in decreased oxygenation.

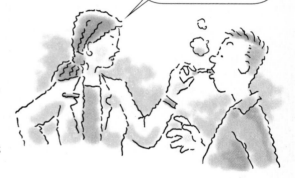

Be sure to explain to your patient ways in which smoking cessation facilitates wound healing.

Pain

In order to promote comfort, you should control the patient's pain to the best of your ability. Pain control also has a practical purpose. In response to pain, the body releases epinephrine, a powerful vasoconstrictor. Vasoconstriction reduces blood flow to the wound. When you relieve pain, vasoconstriction subsides, blood vessels dilate, and blood flow to the wound improves.

Assessing the patient's pain is an important part of wound assessment. You'll want to note pain associated with the injury itself along with pain associated with healing and therapies employed to promote healing. To fully understand the patient's pain, talk with him and ask about his pain. Then, independently, watch to see how he responds to pain and the therapies provided. As always, remember to record your findings. (See *How to assess pain.*)

How to assess pain

To properly assess your patient's pain, consider the patient's descriptions and your own observations of his reaction to pain and treatments.

Talk to your patient

Begin your pain assessment by asking your patient the following questions:

• Where is the pain located? How long does it last? How often does it occur?

• What does the pain feel like? (Let your patient describe it; don't prompt.)

• What relieves the pain? What makes it worse?

• How do you usually get relief?

• How would you rate your pain on a scale of 0 to 10, with 0 representing no pain and 10 representing the worst pain?

Talking with your patient about his pain in this manner helps him define his pain, for himself as well as you, and helps you evaluate the effectiveness of therapies used to relieve pain.

Monitor and observe your patient

As you work with your patient, observe his responses to pain and to interventions intended to relieve pain.

Behavioral responses to watch for include:

• altered body position

• moaning

• sighing

• grimacing

• withdrawing from painful stimuli

• crying

• restlessness

• muscle twitching

• immobility.

Sympathetic responses, normally associated with mild to moderate pain include:

• pallor

• elevated blood pressure

• dilated pupils

• tension in skeletal muscles

• dyspnea (shortness of breath)

• tachycardia (rapid heart beat)

• diaphoresis (sweating).

Parasympathetic responses, which are more common in cases of severe, deep pain include:

• pallor

• lower than normal blood pressure

• bradycardia (slower than normal heartbeat)

• nausea and vomiting

• weakness

• dizziness

• loss of consciousness.

Listen and learn

If the patient is conscious and can communicate, have him rate his pain before and during each dressing change. If your notes reveal that his pain is higher before the dressing change, it may indicate an impending infection, even before any other signs appear.

If the patient says the dressing change itself is painful, you might consider administering pain medication before the procedure or changing the dressing technique itself. For example, if treatment calls for a wet-to-dry debridement technique, you can anticipate that the patient will experience pain and administer preprocedure pain medication accordingly. Remember to document this pain and report it to the practitioner. Less painful methods of removing dead tissue exist but

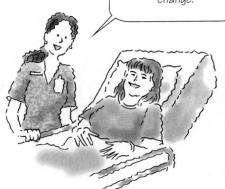

If your patient is able, have her rate her pain before and during each dressing change.

if the patient's pain isn't documented and communicated, wet-to-dry debridement orders may stand and the patient may suffer unnecessary discomfort.

Easy does it

In general, when removing adherent dressings, it's less painful for the patient if you soak the dressing. Over intact skin, you can also use an adhesive remover. Remember to keep the skin taut. Press down on the skin to release the dressing, rather than just pulling the dressing off. If the patient still says that dressing removal is painful, the team may wish to choose a less adherent dressing type.

Cause

Focus on the cause of the wound to help ensure that you consider all factors that can influence healing. For instance, if you're assessing a patient with a venous insufficiency ulcer, you should measure the wound but you should also measure calf circumference regularly to determine if efforts to reduce edema are succeeding. The best interventions for a venous insufficiency ulcer won't heal the wound if edema is left unchecked.

Diabetic details

Similarly, if you're assessing the wound of a patient with diabetes, check to make sure that his blood glucose is well controlled and that the calluses around a diabetic foot ulcer are removed regularly. Otherwise, healing will be impeded.

In other words, as you focus on specific wound characteristics and track the healing process, never lose sight of the big picture.

Assessing the wound bed

Asess the wound bed and the surrounding skin only after they have been cleaned. As you assess the wound bed, record information about:
- dimensions, including length, width, and depth
- tunneling and undermining
- texture
- moisture
- margins and surrounding skin.

Dimensions

Because accurately recording wound dimensions is important, many health care facilities use photography as a tool in wound assessment. If photography is available in your facility, it should be in-

Get wise to wounds

What's missing?

If wound photography is a routine part of your wound documentation system, remember that a picture may be worth a thousand words but your assessment skills and personal observations are still essential. Many wound characteristics can't be recorded accurately—or at all—on film. These include:

- location
- depth
- tunnel measurement
- odor
- feel of surrounding tissue
- pain.

All of this information is needed if the health care team is to make sound treatment decisions.

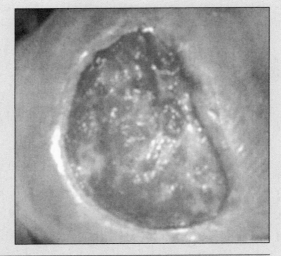

Photograph reprinted with permission from the National Pressure Ulcer Advisory Panel slide series #1. Available: *www.npuap.org*.

cluded in your assessment of wound characteristics. Some photographic techniques produce a picture with a grid overlay that's useful for measuring. Remember, however, that there are qualities of the wound that a camera simply can't record. (See *What's missing?*)

Get out your ruler

The most common method of measuring wound dimensions is to use a tape measure. Make sure it's a disposable device to prevent contamination and cross-contamination. Record the length of the wound as the longest overall distance across the wound (regardless of orientation), and record the width as the longest measurement perpendicular (at a right angle) to your length measurement. (See *Measuring a wound*, page 34.)

Be sure to record any observed areas of intact skin discoloration around the wound opening separately—not as part of the wound bed. Record all measurements in centimeters.

Use a disposable tape measure to measure the length and width of your patient's wound.

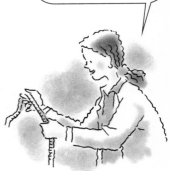

Get wise to wounds

Measuring a wound

When measuring a wound, first determine the longest distance across the open area of the wound—regardless of orientation. In this photo, note the line used to illustrate length.

A wound's width is simply the longest distance across the wound at a right angle to the length. Note the relationship of length and width in this photo. Measure and record areas of reddened, intact skin and white skin as surrounding erythema and maceration—not as part of the wound itself. For a wound like the one in this photo, you would also record a depth and note any areas of tunneling or undermining.

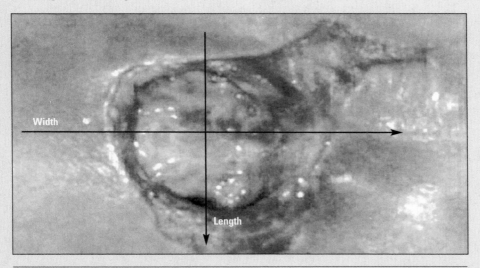

Photograph reprinted with permission from Ayello, E.A. and Baranoski, S. *Wound Care Essentials: Practice Principles.* Philadelphia: Lippincott Williams & Wilkins, 2004.

Just a trace

Another way to measure the wound is to use wound tracing (wound margins are traced on a sheet of clear plastic). You can use the tracing to calculate an approximate wound area. This method provides only a rough estimate but is simple and fairly quick.

How deep

To measure wound depth, you'll need a flexible foam-tipped device. (You may use a cotton-tipped swab but it isn't recommended because the cotton fibers could be left in the wound and the rigid cotton tip may cause trauma to the wound.) Gently insert the device into the deepest portion of the wound and then carefully mark the stick where it meets the edge of the skin. Remove the device and measure the distance from your mark to the end to determine depth. Remember, never probe surgical wounds because they're full-thickness wounds.

Tunneling and undermining

It's also important to measure tunnels, or sinus tracts (extensions of the wound bed into adjacent tissue), and undermining (areas of the wound bed that extend under the skin). Measure tunneling and undermining just as you would wound depth. Carefully insert a flexible foam-tipped device to the bottom of the tunnel or to the end of the undermined area; then mark the stick and measure the distance from your mark to the end of the device. If a tunnel is large, palpate it with a gloved finger rather than a foam-tipped device because you can sense the end of the tunnel better with your finger. This also avoids damaging the tissue.

Texture

The texture of the wound bed provides important information about the wound and how it's healing. If you note very smooth red tissue in a partial-thickness wound, it's most likely the dermis. In a full-thickness wound, it's probably muscle tissue—not granulation tissue. In a full-thickness wound, healthy, red granulation tissue is a sign of proper healing. Healthy granulation tissue has a soft, bumpy appearance.

Moisture

The wound bed should be moist—but not overly moist. Moisture allows the cells and chemicals needed for healing to move about the wound surface.

Desert storm

In dry wound beds, cells involved in healing, which normally exist in a fluid environment, can't move. WBCs can't fight infection, enzymes such as collagenase can't break down dead material, and macrophages can't carry away debris. The wound edges curl up to preserve the moisture that remains in the edge and epithelial cells (new skin cells) fail to grow over and cover the wound. Healing grinds to a halt and necrotic tissue builds up.

Flood watch

Too much moisture poses a different problem. It floods the wound and spills out onto the skin, where the constant moisture causes the death of skin cells.

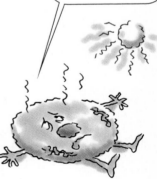

Gasp! Dryness is a drag. If the wound bed is too dry, I can't move. This makes it hard for me to advance healing.

Margins and surrounding skin

When assessing wound margins, you'll want to see skin that's smooth — not rolled — and tightly adherent to the wound bed. Rolled skin may indicate that the wound bed is too dry. Loose skin at the edges may indicate additional shearing injury (separation of skin layers), possibly due to a rough transfer or repositioning. In this case, improve transfer and repositioning techniques to prevent recurrence.

> If your patient's wound is surrounded by white skin, suspect maceration; if you observe red skin, suspect infection.

Rainbow connections

The color of the skin around the wound can alert you to impending problems that can impede healing:
• White skin indicates maceration, or too much moisture, and signals the need for a protective barrier around the wound and a more absorbent dressing.
• Red skin can indicate inflammation, injury (for example, tape burn, excessive pressure, or chemical exposure), or infection. (Remember that inflammation is healthy only during the inflammatory phase of healing.)
• Purple skin can indicate bruising — a sign of trauma.

Let your fingers do the talking

During your assessment of the area around the wound, use your fingers to gain valuable information. For example, gently probe the tissue around the wound bed to determine if it's soft or hard (indurated). Indurated tissue, even in the absence of erythema (redness), is one indication of infection. Similarly, if the patient has dark skin, it may be impossible to see color cues. Again, your fingers can help. Probe the area around the wound bed and compare the feel to surrounding healthy skin. A tender area of skin that appears shiny and feels hard may indicate inflammation.

Assessing drainage

To begin collecting information about wound drainage, inspect the dressing as you remove it and record answers to questions, such as:
• Is the drainage well contained or is it oozing from the edges? If it's oozing, consider using a more absorbent dressing.
• If you're using an occlusive dressing, were the dressing edges well sealed? (A hydrocolloid in the gluteal cleft area becomes a

greenhouse for bacteria if the edges are loose.) If the patient has fecal incontinence, it's even more important to note the seal status.
- Is the dressing saturated or dry?
- How much drainage is there: a scant, moderate, or large amount?
- What are the color and consistency of the drainage? (See *Drainage descriptors*.)
- Is there an odor emanating from the drainage?
- Does the drainage have a thick texture?

Odor

If kept clean, a noninfected wound usually produces little, if any, odor. (One exception is the odor normally present under a hydrocolloid dressing that develops as a by-product of the degradation process.) A newly detected odor might be a sign of infection. Be sure to record odor in your findings and report it to the practitioner. When documenting wound odor, it's important to include when you noted the odor and whether it went away with wound cleaning.

If an odor develops, it can present an embarrassing or otherwise uncomfortable situation for the patient as well as his family, guests, and roommate. If you notice an odor, or if the patient says he notices one, use an odor eliminator. Odor eliminators differ

Get wise to wounds

Drainage descriptors

This chart provides terminology that you can use to describe the color and consistency of wound drainage.

Description	Color and consistency
Serous	• Clear or light yellow • Thin and watery
Sanguineous	• Red (with fresh blood) • Thin
Serosanguineous	• Pink to light red • Thin and watery
Purulent	• Creamy yellow, green, white, or tan • Thick and opaque

from air fresheners because they aren't scents that mask odors but rather compounds that bind with, and neutralize, the molecules responsible for the odor.

Texture

Also consider the texture of the drainage. If the drainage has a thick, creamy texture, the wound contains an excessive amount of bacteria; however, this doesn't necessarily mean a clinically significant infection is present. Document the characteristics of the drainage. Drainage might be creamy because it contains WBCs that have killed bacteria. The drainage is also contaminated with surface bacteria that naturally live in moist environments on the human body. Because of this bacterial colonization, guidelines developed by the Agency for Healthcare Research and Quality recommend against using swab cultures to identify wound infections. However, some practitioners still order swab cultures because they're easy to collect and inexpensive.

Ideally, obtain a swab of the clear fluid expressed from the wound tissue after you've thoroughly cleaned the wound. This is more likely to produce a sample of the bacteria in question. Punch biopsy of tissue or needle aspiration of fluid may also be used. These methods are performed by a doctor or nurse practitioner but will produce more accurate results.

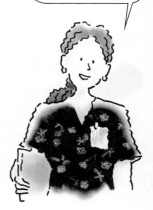

Remember to document the texture of a wound's drainage.

Wound classification

The words you choose to describe your observations of a specific wound have to communicate the same thing to other members of the health care team, insurance companies, regulators, the patient's family and, ultimately, the patient himself. This is a tall order when you consider that even wound care experts debate the descriptive phrases they use. Slough or eschar? Undermining or tunneling? How much drainage is "moderate"? Is the color green or yellow?

The best way to classify wounds is to use the basic system described here, which focuses on three categories of fundamental characteristics:

- type
- age
- depth.

Type

Two basic types of wounds exist: surgical and nonsurgical. A surgical wound is caused by a surgical procedure. A nonsurgical

Get wise to wounds

Tailoring wound care to wound assessment

Wound bed condition	Management techniques
Granulation tissue	• Cover the wound to keep it clean and protected. Keep the wound moist. • For minimal drainage, use a transparent film, hydrocolloid, or hydrogel dressing. • Absorb drainage by using foams, alginates, or hydrofibers. • Remember, beefy red may indicate bioburden of the wound bed and a topical antimicrobial may be warranted (silver, cadexomer iodine).
Fibrin slough	• Debride the wound using enzymatic debridement or pulsatile lavage. • Use a moisture retentive dressing to stimulate autolytic debridement, such as transparent films, hydrocolloids, or hydrogels. • Use an alginate or Hydrofiber to absorb drainage and support autolytic debridement. • Topical antimicrobials may also be indicated in this wound.
Eschar	• Depending on the location, use conservative sharp or enzymatic (Accuzyme or Gladase) debridement or pulsatile lavage methods. • Keep wounds with inadequate blood supply and noninfected heel ulcers clean and dry. • Topical antimicrobials may also be indicated in this wound as the tissue begins to break down.

wound can be caused by trauma or may be a pressure ulcer, diabetic foot ulcer, or vascular ulcer. (See *Tailoring wound care to wound assessment*.)

Age

When determining wound age, you need to first determine if the wound is acute or chronic. However, this determination can present a problem if you adhere solely to a timeline. For instance, just how long is it before an acute wound becomes a chronic wound?

A different way of thinking

Rather than base your determination solely on time, consider a wound acute if it's new or making progress as expected. Consider a wound chronic if it isn't healing in a timely fashion. The main idea is that, in a chronic wound, healing has slowed or stopped and the wound is no longer getting smaller and shallower. Even if the wound bed appears healthy, red, and moist, if healing fails to progress, consider it a chronic wound.

More bad than good

Chronic wounds don't heal as easily as acute wounds. The drainage in chronic wounds contains a greater amount of destructive enzymes, and fibroblasts (the cells that function as the architects in wound healing) seem to lose their "oomph." They're less effective at producing collagen, divide less often, and send fewer signals to other cells telling them to divide and fill the wound. In other words, the wound changes from one that's vigorous and ready to heal, to one that's downright lazy!

Depth

Depth is another fundamental characteristic used to classify wounds. In your assessment, record wound depth as partial-thickness or full-thickness. (See *Classifying wound depth.*)

Get wise to wounds

Classifying wound depth

A wound is classified as partial-thickness or full-thickness according to its depth. Partial-thickness wounds involve only the epidermis or extend into the dermis but not through it. Full-thickness wounds extend through the dermis into tissues beneath and may expose adipose tissue, muscle, or bone. These diagrams illustrate the relative depth of both classifications.

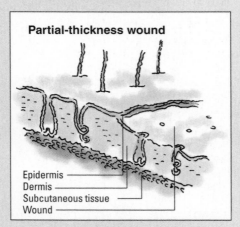

Partial-thickness wound

Epidermis
Dermis
Subcutaneous tissue
Wound

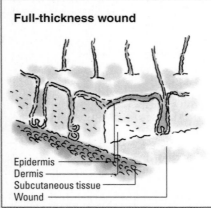

Full-thickness wound

Epidermis
Dermis
Subcutaneous tissue
Wound

Partial-thickness

Partial-thickness wounds normally heal quickly because they involve only the epidermal layer of the skin or extend through the epidermis into (but not through) the dermis. The dermis remains at least partially intact to generate the new epidermis needed to close the wound. Partial-thickness wounds are also less susceptible to infection because part of the body's first level of defense (partial dermis) is still intact. These wounds tend to be painful, however, and need protection from the air to reduce pain.

Full-thickness

Full-thickness wounds penetrate completely through the skin into underlying tissues. The wound may expose adipose tissue (fat), muscle, tendon, or bone. In the abdomen, you may see adipose tissue or omentum (the covering of the bowel). If the omentum is penetrated, the bowel may protrude through the wound (evisceration). Granulation tissue may be visible if the wound has started to heal.

Full-thickness wounds heal by granulation and contraction, which require more body resources and more time than the healing of partial-thickness wounds. When assessing a full-thickness wound, report its depth as well as its length and width.

The added pressure of pressure ulcers

In the case of pressure ulcers, wound depth allows you to stage the ulcer according to the classification system developed by the National Pressure Ulcer Advisory Panel (NPUAP). (See chapter 6, Pressure ulcers.)

Wound monitoring

Monitor the patient throughout the healing process, periodically reassessing his status and documenting his progress toward full healing. Wound monitoring is a requirement for some regulatory agencies such as the Centers for Medicare and Medicaid Services (CMS).

Paint a picture

Your initial assessment sets the benchmark for subsequent monitoring and reassessment activities. One assessment is a static report; a series of assessments, however, can illustrate the dynamic aspect of the healing process. In this way, all members of the health care team can see the patient's progress toward healing (or failure

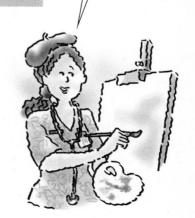

The picture of the wound that you paint during your initial assessment plays an important role in wound monitoring.

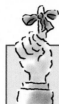

Memory jogger

Use the mnemonic device WOUND PICTURE to help you recall and organize key facts in your documentation:

Wound or ulcer location

Odor (in the room or after uncovering the wound)

Ulcer category, stage (for pressure ulcer) or classification (for diabetic ulcer), and depth (partial-thickness or full-thickness)

Necrotic tissue

Dimension (shape, length, width, depth); drainage color, consistency, and amount (scant, moderate, large)

Pain (when it occurs, what relieves it, patient's description, and patient's rating on scale of 0 to 10)

Induration (hard or soft surrounding tissue)

Color of wound bed (red-yellow-black or combination)

Tunneling (length and direction — toward patient's right, left, head, feet)

Undermining (length and direction, using clock references to describe)

Redness or other discoloration in surrounding skin

Edge of skin loose or tightly adhered and edges flat or rolled under

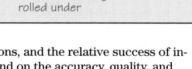

to heal), developing complications, and the relative success of interventions. The view will depend on the accuracy, quality, and consistency of your documentation.

In the course of a wound assessment, you amass quite a bit of useful information about the patient, his environment, the characteristics of his wound, and his current status in the healing process. When documenting your assessment, be sure to include the date and time of your observations. Also, strive to obtain accurate measurements, using appropriate units of measurement. Make sure that the entire health care team is using the same tool to measure the patient's wound. Remember to document only the facts, not your opinions about the wound.

The prospect of monitoring, reassessing, and documenting over time may seem daunting; however, several research-based documentation tools are available — or your facility may have its own tool — to help you manage the task.

Documentation tools

Most wound documentation tools in use in the United States focus on pressure ulcers. Pressure ulcers were selected because of their tremendous impact on countless patients' lives and the health care system itself. Pressure ulcers are painful, typically chronic, life-disrupting, and expensive to treat — both in dollars and in amount of time spent by providers — and are usually preventable.

Pressure Ulcer Scale for Healing

The Pressure Ulcer Scale for Healing (PUSH) tool was developed and revised by the NPUAP and is only applicable to pressure ulcers. It's simple, quick, and easy to score. (See *PUSH tool*, page 44.)

When working with this tool, you develop three scores: one for the surface area (length × width), one for the drainage amount, and one for the tissue type in the wound during each review. The sum of these scores yields a total score for the wound on a given day. This score is then plotted on a pressure ulcer healing record and healing graph. By recording and reviewing scores over time, you can determine the pace of progress toward healing.

The NPUAP is working with CMS to incorporate the PUSH tool into resident assessment protocols to accompany the Minimum Data Set in long-term care facilities.

Pressure Sore Status Tool

The Pressure Sore Status Tool (PSST) allows you to track scores for 11 factors over time. These factors are each scored based on a number scale, and the scores are added. The total score reflects overall wound status.

The PSST is a precise record of wound changes and is fairly time consuming to fill out. Consequently, it's used more in research than in clinical practice.

Wound Healing Scale

The Wound Healing Scale is a simple classification system that combines a designation for wound stage, or thickness, with a tissue descriptor. For example, a stage III pressure ulcer containing necrotic tissue is recorded as 3N. Using this tool, you can track the general direction of healing by noting, for example, that this week the wound is an FG (full-thickness with granulation tissue), whereas last week it was an FN (full-thickness with necrotic tissue). The tool includes modifiers that permit you to use it for all types of wounds, although it was developed initially for use with pressure ulcers.

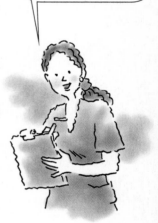

Use the PUSH tool for a quick and easy way to document pressure ulcer healing.

PUSH tool

The Pressure Ulcer Scale for Healing (PUSH) tool is simple to use and quick and easy to score.

Patient name _Doris McCoy_   User location _Rockdale Nursing Home_

Patient I.D. # _0162386_   Date _7/26/06_

Directions

Observe and measure the pressure ulcer. Categorize the ulcer with respect to surface area, exudate, and type of wound tissue. Record a subscore for each of the ulcer characteristics. Add the subscores to obtain the total score. A comparison of total scores measured over time provides an indication of the improvement or deterioration in pressure ulcer healing.

Length × width	0	1	2	3	4	5	Subscore
	0 cm²	< 0.3 cm²	0.3 to 0.6 cm²	(0.7 to 1 cm²)	1.1 to 2 cm²	2.1 to 3 cm²	3
	6	7	8	9	10		
	3.1 to 4 cm²	4.1 to 8 cm²	8.1 to 12 cm²	12.1 to 24 cm²	> 24 cm²		

Exudate amount	0	1	2	3			Subscore
	None	Light	(Moderate)	Heavy			2

Tissue type	0	1	2	3	4		Subscore
	Closed	(Epithelial tissue)	Granulation tissue	Slough	Necrotic tissue		1

Total score: 6

Length × width

Measure the greatest length (head-to-toe) and the greatest width (side-to-side) using a centimeter ruler. Multiply these two measurements (length × width) to obtain an estimate of surface area in square centimeters (cm²). Don't guess! Always use a centimeter ruler and always use the same method each time the ulcer is measured.

Exudate amount

Estimate the amount of exudate (drainage) present after removing the dressing and before applying any topical agent to the ulcer. Estimate the exudate as none, light, moderate, or heavy.

Tissue type

This refers to the types of tissue that are present in the wound (ulcer) bed. Score as a 4 if you note necrotic tissue. Score as a 3 if you observe slough but no necrotic tissue. Score as a 2 if the wound is clean and contains granulation tissue. Score a superficial wound that's reepithelializing as a 1. When the wound is closed, score it as a 0. The following guidelines describe each tissue type:

4 — Necrotic tissue (eschar): Black, brown, or tan tissue that adheres firmly to the wound bed or ulcer edges and may be either firmer or softer than surrounding tissue

3 — Slough: Yellow or white tissue that adheres to the ulcer bed in strings or thick clumps or is mucinous

2 — Granulation tissue: Pink or beefy red tissue with a shiny, moist, granular appearance

1 — Epithelial tissue: For superficial ulcers, new pink or shiny tissue (skin) that grows in from the edges or as islands on the ulcer surface

0 — Closed or resurfaced: Completely covered wound with epithelium (new skin)

Adapted with permission from PUSH tool version 3.0, © 1998 National Pressure Ulcer Advisory Panel, Reston, Va.

Sussman Wound Healing Tool

The Sussman Wound Healing Tool was developed to help physical therapists track pressure ulcer healing. This tool lists 10 wound attributes and classifies each as "good" or "not good" in terms of wound healing. For example, granulation tissue is classified "good" and undermining is classified "not good." During each assessment, record your findings for each of the 10 attributes that apply to the patient; over time, this provides a picture of wound healing or failure to heal.

> In wound care, you may be able to foresee problems by recognizing signs of complications or failure to heal.

Recognizing complications

It's important to monitor and track, or reassess, wound status to identify signs and symptoms of complications or failure to heal as early in the process as possible. Early intervention improves the likelihood of resolving complications successfully and getting the healing process back on track.

Oh say, can you see?

You'll conduct your reassessments using the same criteria used in the initial assessment, with one added advantage — perspective. Careful monitoring can help you catch failure to heal early so you can intervene appropriately. (See *Recognizing failure to heal*, pages 46 and 47.)

The sooner, the better

Success or failure of the healing process has a tremendous impact on the patient's quality of life as well as his family's quality of life. Early intervention can mean that a patient with a diabetic foot ulcer can avoid amputation or a paraplegic patient with an ischial ulcer can once again sit up and lead an active life.

Chronic ulcers pose a particularly difficult problem, not only for individual practitioners but also for the health care industry as a whole. Treating chronic ulcers is expensive because they're difficult or impossible to heal. Consequently, the people responsible for the largest portion of the bill — the government and insurance companies — are placing increased emphasis on early intervention and prevention.

Winning in wound healing

Now that you know what to look for when things *aren't* going well, let's take a look at what you can expect to see when healing is progressing smoothly. In this case, the patient:
• is well hydrated, well nourished, comfortable, and warm

Get wise to wounds

Recognizing failure to heal

This chart presents the most common signs of failure to heal as well as associated probable causes and appropriate interventions.

Sign	Causes	Interventions
Wound bed		
Too dry	• Exposure of tissue and cells normally in a moist environment to air • Inadequate hydration	• Add moisture regularly. • Use a dressing that maintains moisture, such as a transparent film, hydrocolloid, or hydrogel dressing.
No change in size or depth for 2 weeks	• Pressure or trauma to the area • Poor nutrition, poor circulation, or inadequate hydration • Poor control of disease processes such as diabetes • Inadequate pain control • Infection • Debridement	• Reassess the patient for local or systemic problems that impair wound healing, and intervene as necessary. • If caused by debridement, no intervention is necessary.
Increase in size or depth	• Ischemia due to excess pressure or poor circulation • Infection	• Poor circulation may not be resolvable, but consider adding warmth to the area and administering a vasodilator or antiplatelet medication. Address possible infection.
Necrosis	• Ischemia	• Perform debridement if the remaining living tissue has adequate circulation.
Increase in drainage or change of drainage color from clear to purulent	• Autolytic or enzymatic debridement • Infection	• If caused by autolytic or enzymatic debridement, no intervention is necessary. An increase in drainage or change of drainage color is expected because of the breakdown of dead tissue. • If debridement isn't the cause, assess the wound for infection.
Tunneling	• Pressure over bony prominences • Presence of foreign body • Deep infection	• Protect the area from pressure. • Irrigate and inspect the tunnel as carefully as possible for a hidden suture or leftover bit of dressing material. • If the tunnel doesn't shorten in length each week, thoroughly clean and obtain a tissue biopsy for infection and, with a chronic wound, for possible malignancy.

Recognizing failure to heal (continued)

Sign	Causes	Interventions
Wound edges		
Red, hot skin; tenderness; and induration	• Inflammation due to excess pressure or infection	• Protect the area from pressure. • If pressure relief doesn't resolve the inflammation within 24 hours, topical antimicrobial therapy may be indicated.
Maceration (white skin)	• Excess moisture	• Protect the skin with petrolatum ointment or barrier wipe. • If practical, obtain an order for a more absorptive dressing.
Rolled skin edges	• Too-dry wound bed	• Obtain an order for moisture-retentive dressings. • If rolling isn't resolved in 1 week, debridement of the edges may be necessary.
Undermining or ecchymosis of surrounding skin (loose or bruised skin edges)	• Excess shearing force to the area	• Initiate measures to protect the area, especially during patient transfers.

• is well managed for associated or contributing diseases, such as diabetes, heart failure, or renal failure
• exhibits normal immune system response.
   In addition, the wound itself:
• receives the oxygen and nutrients it needs (adequate vascular supply)
• is moist and protected from the environment
• is free from necrotic tissue.
   These conditions optimize wound healing. By using the assessment techniques presented in this chapter, you'll be a part of this success.

Star player

Wound healing isn't a simple matter to coordinate. Through vigilance and consistent assessment and documentation, success is much more likely. By using most of your senses, you can have a tremendous influence on whether a wound heals or becomes chronic and harder to manage. Recognizing red flags that warn of failure to heal, and knowing the appropriate interventions, make you a part of the winning wound healing team!

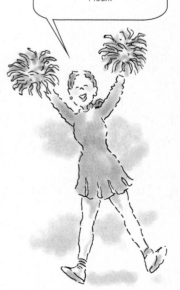

Give me an H! Give me an E! Give me an A! Give me an L! What does that spell? Heal!

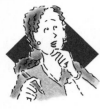

Quick quiz

1. A wound that extends through the epidermis and part way into the dermis is classified as a:

    A.   chronic wound.

    B.   acute wound.

    C.   partial-thickness wound.

    D.   full-thickness wound.

Answer: C. Partial-thickness wounds extend into but not through the dermis, which retains function that helps the healing process.

2. Which wound bed color indicates normal, healthy granulation tissue?

    A.   Red

    B.   Yellow

    C.   Tan

    D.   Black

Answer: A. Red tissue in a wound bed indicates healthy granulation tissue.

3. If you see multiple colors in a wound bed, you should describe the wound according to the:

    A.   percentage of tissue types.

    B.   least healthy color you see.

    C.   color most visible.

    D.   least percentage of tissue.

Answer: A. Describe a wound with multiple colors according to the percentage of tissue types in the wound bed.

4. Wound healing is facilitated by:

    A.   a dark environment.

    B.   exposure to air.

    C.   a dry environment.

    D.   a moist environment.

Answer: D. Moisture in the wound bed allows the cells and chemicals needed for healing to move across the wound surface.

5. The PUSH tool is useful for:
  A. measuring the size of a pressure ulcer.
  B. detecting wound infection.
  C. tracking pressure ulcer healing.
  D. measuring the depth of a pressure ulcer.

Answer: C. The PUSH tool allows you to track pressure ulcer healing.

6. Which term could be used to accurately describe drainage that's thin and bright red?
  A. Serous
  B. Sanguineous
  C. Serosanguineous
  D. Purulent

Answer: B. Sanguineous drainage is red, usually due to the presence of fresh blood.

7. Which is an appropriate intervention for a wound that has tunneling?
  A. Provide warmth to the area.
  B. Perform conservative sharp debridement.
  C. Protect the area from pressure.
  D. No intervention is necessary.

Answer: C. Because tunneling may be caused by pressure over bony prominences, the wound should be protected from

8. What would your assessment of a nonhealing would show if the cause was a too-dry wound bed?
  A. Rolled skin edges
  B. Maceration
  C. Red, hot skin
  D. Undermining

Answer: A. A wound bed that's too dry exhibits rolled skin edges and requires moisture-retentive dressings or debridement.

Scoring

☆☆☆   If you answered all eight questions correctly, stand up and bow!
You're a wound care all-star.

☆☆   If you answered five to seven questions correctly, great job!
You're a cut above the rest.

☆   If you answered fewer than five questions correctly, don't worry!
You've just skinned the surface of wound care; there are nine
more chapters to go.

3

Basic wound care procedures

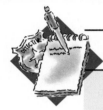

Just the facts

In this chapter, you'll learn:

♦ components of a wound care order

♦ wound cleaning and irrigation techniques

♦ dressing application techniques

♦ debridement techniques

♦ specimen collection techniques.

A look at wound care orders

Wound care orders are typically written by doctors, podiatrists, nurse practitioners, and physician's assistants. However, policies and procedures related to skin and wound care activities are commonly written and carried out by registered nurses with the doctor in charge of reviewing and approving them. Many facilities now have specific policies and procedures for different types of wounds.

Make sure that your wound care orders contain all the necessary information.

What to include

When you're presented with an order to provide wound care, or if you're in the position to write wound policies and procedures, keep in mind the following list of essential information that you should include:

• wound description, including cause, location, appearance, and size

• cleaning agent and method to be used

• type of dressing for the primary and, if needed, secondary layers

• topical medications needed

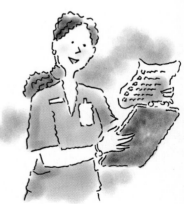

- frequency of dressing changes
- time frame for evaluating and changing dressings.

Typically, if there's no change in the wound in 2 weeks, the patient's condition and wound should be reassessed and the management plan should be revised accordingly. New orders may be needed. If no healing progress is apparent after 4 to 12 weeks of treatment, referral to a wound care specialist is recommended.

Determining a wound care plan

Wound care is based on the whole patient: his condition, his needs, and the wound profile. The goals of wound care include:
- promoting wound healing by controlling or eliminating causative factors
- preventing or managing infection
- removing nonviable tissue (debridement) as needed
- enhancing adequate blood supply
- providing nutritional and fluid support
- establishing and maintaining a clean, moist, protected wound bed
- managing wound fluid or drainage
- maintaining the skin surrounding the wound to ensure that it remains dry and intact.

With any wound, promote healing by keeping the wound moist, clean, and free from debris. However, requirements for providing wound care vary according to the patient assessment and the nature of the wound. (See *Guide to making wound care decisions*.)

Basic wound care

Basic wound care centers on cleaning and dressing the wound. Because open wounds are colonized (or contaminated) with bacteria, observe clean technique using clean, nonsterile gloves during wound care unless sterile dressing changes are specified. Always follow standard precautions.

Clean machine

The goal of wound cleaning is to remove debris and contaminants from the wound without damaging healthy tissue. The wound should be cleaned initially; repeat cleaning as needed or with each dressing change.

Dress to impress

The basic purpose of a dressing is to provide an optimal environment in which the body can heal itself. Consider this environment

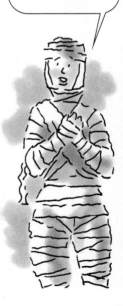

No need to keep it under wraps. Everyone should know that basic wound care involves cleaning and dressing the wound.

Get wise to wounds

Guide to making wound care decisions

Ask yourself the following questions to help you determine what kind of care your patient's wound needs and how you should proceed. Make sure you assess the wound and document according to your facility's policy and procedure.

How should I clean the wound?
___ Water ___ Saline ___ Commercial wound cleaner

Is the wound partial-thickness or full-thickness?
___ Partial ___ Full

Is the wound clean, necrotic, or infected?
___ Clean ___ Necrotic ___ Infected

Is gangrene present?
___ Yes ___ No

Is there blood flow to the area?
___ Yes ___ No

Does the wound need debridement?
___ Yes ___ No

What kind of debridement is appropriate?
___ Sharp ___ Chemical ___ Mechanical ___ Autolytic

How much drainage is present?
___ None ___ Minimal ___ Moderate ___ Heavy

How does the surrounding skin appear?
___ Intact ___ Irritated ___ Denuded

What cover or dressing is appropriate?
___ Transparent film ___ Hydrogel ___ Hydrocolloid ___ Alginate ___ Foam
___ Gauze ___ Other

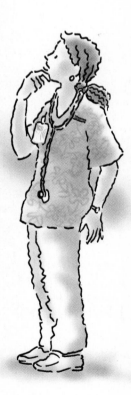

before you select a dressing. Functions of a wound dressing include:

- protecting the wound from contamination and trauma
- providing compression if bleeding or swelling is anticipated
- applying medications
- absorbing drainage or debrided necrotic tissue
- filling or packing the wound
- protecting the skin surrounding the wound.

Follow the golden rule

The cardinal rule is to keep wound tissue moist and surrounding tissue dry. Ideally, a dressing should keep the wound moist, absorb drainage or debris, conform to the wound, and be adhesive to surrounding skin yet also be easily removable. It should also be user-friendly, require minimal changes, decrease the need for a secondary dressing layer, and be cost-effective and comfortable for the patient.

What you need

Hypoallergenic tape or elastic netting ❋ overbed table ❋ piston-type irrigating system ❋ two pairs of clean or sterile gloves (depending on facility policy) ❋ cleaning solution (such as normal saline solution) as ordered ❋ clean or sterile bowl (depending on facility policy) ❋ sterile 4″ × 4″ gauze pads ❋ selected topical dressing ❋ linen-saver pads ❋ impervious plastic trash bag ❋ disposable wound-measuring device ❋ sterile flexible foam-tipped devices

Getting ready

Confirm the patient's identity using two patient identifiers according to your facility's policy. Then assemble the equipment at the patient's bedside. Use clean or sterile technique, depending on your facility's policy and wound care orders. Cut tape into strips for securing dressings. Loosen lids on cleaning solutions and medications for easy removal. Attach an impervious plastic trash bag to the overbed table to hold used dressings and refuse.

How you do it

Before any dressing change, wash your hands and review the principles of standard precautions.

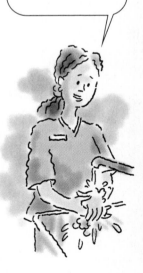

Before any dressing change, be sure to wash your hands. Always follow standard precautions during the procedure.

Get wise to wounds

Choosing a cleaning agent

The most commonly used cleaning agent is sterile normal saline solution, which provides a moist environment, promotes granulation tissue formation, and causes minimal fluid shifts in healthy adults.

Antiseptic solutions may damage tissue and delay healing but are sometimes used for cleaning infected or newly contaminated wounds. Examples of antiseptic solutions include:
• *hydrogen peroxide* (commonly used half-strength), which is used to irrigate the wound and aid in mechanical debridement; its foaming action also warms the wound, promoting vasodilation and reducing inflammation (*Note:* Don't use this solution in surgical wounds.)
• *acetic acid,* which is used to treat *Pseudomonas* infection (*Note:* This solution changes the color of wound drainage.)
• *sodium hypochlorite* (Dakin's fluid), an antiseptic that slightly dissolves necrotic tissue (*Note:* This unstable solution must be freshly prepared every 24 hours.)
• *povidone-iodine,* a broad-spectrum, fast-acting antimicrobial agent. (Watch for patient sensitivity to this solution; also, protect the surrounding skin from contact because this solution can dry and stain the skin.)

Cleaning the wound

• Provide privacy and explain the procedure to the patient to allay his fears and promote cooperation.
• Position the patient in a way that maximizes his comfort while allowing easy access to the wound site.
• Cover bed linens with a linen-saver pad to prevent soiling.

No splashing

• Open the cleaning solution container and carefully pour cleaning solution into a bowl, avoiding splashing. (See *Choosing a cleaning agent.*)
• Open the packages of supplies.
• Put on the first pair of gloves.
• Gently roll or lift an edge of the soiled dressing to obtain a starting point. Support adjacent skin while gently releasing the soiled dressing from the skin. When possible, remove the dressing in the direction of hair growth.
• Discard the soiled dressing and your contaminated gloves in the impervious plastic trash bag to avoid contaminating the clean or sterile field. Then wash your hands.
• Put on a clean pair of gloves.
• Inspect the wound. Note the color, amount, and odor of drainage and necrotic debris.

- Inspect the skin around the wound for redness, heat, and moisture.
- Fold a sterile 4″ × 4″ gauze pad into quarters and grasp it with your fingers. Make sure the folded edge faces outward.
- Dip the folded gauze into the cleaning solution. Or, use a spray gun bottle to apply the solution to the gauze.

Wax on, wax off

- When cleaning, be sure to move from the least-contaminated area to the most-contaminated area. For a linear shaped wound, such as an incision, gently wipe from top to bottom in one motion, starting directly over the wound and moving outward. For an open wound, such as a pressure ulcer, gently wipe in concentric circles, again starting directly over the wound and moving outward.
- Discard the used gauze pad in the plastic trash bag.
- Using a clean gauze pad for each wiping motion, repeat the procedure until you've cleaned the entire wound.
- Dry the wound with 4″ × 4″ gauze pads, using the same procedure as for cleaning. Discard the used gauze pads in the plastic trash bag and then rewash your hands.
- Measure the perimeter of the wound with a disposable wound-measuring device (for example, a square, transparent card with concentric circles arranged in bull's-eye fashion and bordered with a straight-edge ruler). Know your facility's policy for wound measurement and always be consistent in your measurements.
- Measure the depth of a full-thickness wound. Gently insert a sterile flexible foam-tipped device into the deepest part of the wound bed and place a mark on the stick where it meets the skin level. Measure the marked device to determine wound depth.

Testing for tunneling

- Gently probe the wound bed and edges with your finger or with a sterile flexible foam-tipped device to assess for wound tunneling or undermining. Tunneling usually signals wound extension along fascial planes. Gauge tunnel depth by determining how far you can insert your finger or the foam-tipped device.
- Next, reassess the condition of the skin and wound. Note the character of the clean wound bed and the surrounding skin.
- If you observe adherent necrotic material, notify a wound care specialist or a practitioner to ensure appropriate debridement.
- Prepare to apply the appropriate topical dressing. Instructions for applying topical moist saline gauze, hydrocolloid, transparent film, alginate, foam, and hydrogel dressings follow. (See *Choosing a wound dressing.*)

This tunnel sure is deep! When testing for wound tunneling, remember to gently probe the wound bed.

Dress for success

Choosing a wound dressing

The patient's needs and wound characteristics determine which type of dressing you'll use on a wound.

Gauze dressings
Made of absorptive cotton or synthetic fabric, gauze dressings are permeable to water, water vapor, and oxygen and may be impregnated with hydrogel or another agent. When uncertain about which dressing to use, you may apply a gauze dressing moistened in saline solution until a wound specialist recommends definitive treatment.

Hydrocolloid dressings
Hydrocolloid dressings are adhesive, moldable wafers made of a carbohydrate-based material that usually have waterproof backings. They're impermeable to oxygen, water, and water vapor, and most have some absorptive properties.

Transparent film dressings
Transparent film dressings are clear, adherent, and nonabsorptive. These polymer-based dressings are permeable to oxygen and water vapor but not to water. Their transparency allows visual inspection. Because they can't absorb drainage, they're used on partial-thickness wounds with minimal exudate.

Alginate dressings
Made from seaweed, alginate dressings are nonwoven, absorptive dressings available as soft white sterile pads or ropes. They absorb excessive exudate and may be used on infected wounds. As these dressings absorb exudate, they turn into a gel that keeps the wound bed moist and promotes healing. When exudate is no longer excessive, switch to another type of dressing.

Foam dressings
Foam dressings are spongelike polymer dressings that may be impregnated or coated with other materials. Somewhat absorptive, they may be adherent. These dressings promote moist wound healing and are useful when a nonadherent surface is desired.

Hydrogel dressings
Water-based and nonadherent, hydrogel dressings are polymer-based dressings that have some absorptive properties. They're used when the wound needs moisture. Available as a gel in a tube, as flexible sheets, and as saturated gauze packing strips, they may have a cooling effect.

For other dressings or topical agents, follow your facility's protocol or the manufacturer's instructions.

Applying a moist saline gauze dressing
• Moisten the dressing with normal saline solution. Wring out excess fluid.
• Gently place the dressing onto the wound surface. To separate surfaces within the wound, gently guide the gauze between opposing wound surfaces. Don't pack the gauze tightly to avoid damage to tissues.
• Apply a sealant or barrier to protect the surrounding skin from moisture.
• Change the dressing often enough to keep the wound moist.

Applying a hydrocolloid dressing

• Choose a clean, dry, presized dressing, or cut one to overlap the wound by about 1″ (2.5 cm). Remove the dressing from its package, pull the release paper from the adherent side of the dressing, and apply the dressing to the wound. Hold the dressing in place with your hand (the warmth will mold the dressing to the skin).

Smooth operator

• As you apply the dressing, carefully smooth out wrinkles and avoid stretching the dressing.
• If the dressing's edges need to be secured with tape, apply a skin sealant to the intact skin around the wound. After the area dries, tape the dressing to the skin. The sealant protects the skin from tape burns and skin stripping and promotes tape adherence. Avoid using tension or pressure when you apply the tape.
• Remove your gloves and discard them in the impervious plastic trash bag. Dispose of refuse according to your facility's policy and then wash your hands.
• Change a hydrocolloid dressing every 2 to 7 days as necessary; change it immediately if the patient complains of pain, the dressing no longer adheres, or leakage occurs.

Carefully smooth out wrinkles as you apply the dressing to minimize irritation.

Applying a transparent film dressing

• Select a dressing to overlap the wound by 1″ to 2″ (2.5 to 5 cm).
• Gently lay the dressing over the wound; avoid wrinkling the dressing. To prevent shearing force, don't stretch the dressing over the wound. Press firmly on the edges of the dressing to promote adherence. Although this type of dressing is self-adhesive, you may have to tape the edges to prevent them from curling.
• Change the dressing every 3 to 5 days, depending on the amount of drainage. If the seal is no longer secure or if accumulated tissue fluid extends beyond the edges of the wound and onto the surrounding skin, change the dressing.

Applying an alginate dressing

• Apply the dressing to the wound surface. Cover the area with a secondary dressing (such as gauze pads or transparent film), as ordered. Secure the dressing with tape or elastic netting.
• If the wound is draining heavily, change the dressing once or twice daily for the first 3 to 5 days. As drainage decreases, change the dressing less frequently—every 2 to 4 days or as ordered. When the drainage stops or the wound bed looks dry, stop using an alginate dressing.

Applying a foam dressing

- Gently lay the dressing over the wound.
- Use tape, elastic netting, or gauze to hold the dressing in place.
- Change the dressing when the foam no longer absorbs exudate.

Applying a hydrogel dressing

- Apply a moderate amount of gel to the wound bed.
- Cover the area with a secondary dressing (gauze, transparent film, or foam).
- Change the dressing daily or as needed to keep the wound bed moist.
- If the hydrogel dressing you select comes in sheet form, cut the dressing to overlap the wound by 1″; then apply it as you would a hydrocolloid dressing.
- Hydrogel dressings also come as a prepackaged, saturated gauze for wounds with cavities that require filling "dead space." Follow the manufacturer's directions to apply these dressings.

Practice pointers

Be aware that infection may cause foul-smelling drainage, persistent pain, severe erythema, induration, and elevated skin and body temperatures. (However, some dressings and topical agents may also cause an odor.) Advancing infection or cellulitis can lead to septicemia. Severe erythema may signal worsening cellulitis, which means the offending organisms have invaded the tissue and are no longer localized.

Wound irrigation

Irrigation cleans tissues and flushes cell debris and drainage from an open wound. It also helps prevent premature surface healing over an abscess pocket or infected tract.

After irrigation, pack open wounds to absorb additional drainage. Remember to always follow standard precautions.

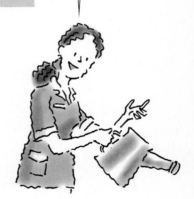

Irrigation cleans tissues and gently flushes away cell debris from an open wound.

What you need

Impervious plastic trash bag ❉ linen-saver pad ❉ emesis basin ❉ two pairs of clean or sterile gloves (depending on facility policy) ❉ protective eyewear, if indicated ❉

gown, if indicated ❊ prescribed irrigant, such as sterile normal saline solution or sterile water ❊ clean or sterile container (depending on facility policy) ❊ materials as needed for wound care ❊ sterile irrigation and dressing set ❊ commercial wound cleaner ❊ 35-ml piston syringe with 19G needle or catheter or commercial wound irrigation set ❊ skin protectant wipe (skin sealant) or other protective skin barrier

Getting ready

Confirm the patient's identity using two patient identifiers according to your facility's policy. Then assemble the equipment in the patient's room. Check the expiration date on each sterile package and inspect the packages for tears.

Don't use any solution that has been open longer than 24 hours. As needed, dilute the prescribed irrigant to the correct proportions with sterile water or normal saline solution. Allow the solution to reach room temperature or warm it to 90° to 95° F (32.2° to 35° C).

Open the waterproof trash bag; place it near the patient's bed. Form a cuff by turning down the top of the trash bag.

How you do it

• Check the practitioner's order, assess the patient's condition, and identify allergies.
• Explain the procedure to the patient, provide privacy, and position the patient correctly for the procedure.
• Place the linen-saver pad under the patient and place the emesis basin below the wound so that the irrigating solution flows from the wound into the basin.
• Wash your hands and then put on a gown and gloves.
• Remove the soiled dressing; then discard the dressing and gloves in the trash bag.
• Establish a clean or sterile field with all the equipment and supplies you'll need for wound irrigation and dressing.
• Pour the prescribed amount of irrigating solution into a clean or sterile container.
• Put on a new pair of gloves and a gown and protective eyewear, if indicated.

From clean to dirty

• Fill the syringe with the irrigating solution and connect the catheter to the syringe.
• Gently instill a slow, steady stream of solution into the wound until the syringe empties. (See *Irrigating a deep wound.*) Make

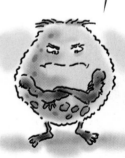

If you aren't careful during irrigation, my pathogenic friends and I will run rampant.

Get wise to wounds

Irrigating a deep wound

When preparing to irrigate a wound, attach a 19G needle or catheter to a 35-ml piston syringe. This setup delivers an irrigation pressure of 8 psi, which will effectively clean the wound and reduce the risk of trauma and wound infection. To prevent tissue damage or, in an abdominal wound, intestinal perforation, avoid forcing the needle or catheter into the wound.

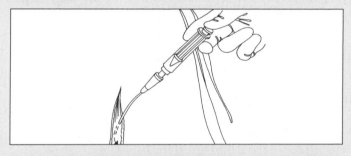

Irrigate the wound with gentle pressure until you've administered the prescribed amount and the solution returns clear. Keep the emesis basin under the wound to collect any remaining drainage.

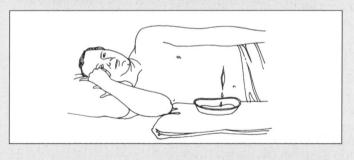

sure the solution flows from the clean to the dirty area of the wound to prevent contamination of clean tissue by exudate. Also make sure the solution reaches all areas of the wound.

• Refill the syringe, reconnect it to the catheter, and repeat the irrigation. Continue to irrigate the wound until you've administered the prescribed amount of solution or until the solution returns clear. Note the amount of solution administered. Then remove and discard the catheter and syringe in the waterproof trash bag. (See *Wound irrigation tips*, page 62.)

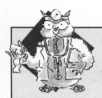

Get wise to wounds

Wound irrigation tips

How can you avoid mess or spillage when irrigating a wound in a hard-to-reach location? Here are some tips you can follow.

Limb wounds

You can soak an arm or a leg wound in a large vessel of warm irrigating fluid, such as water, normal saline solution, or an appropriate antiseptic. An agitator can help dislodge bacteria and loosen debris. Remember that this method is contraindicated in patient's with cellulitis, unstable coagulation studies, or deep vein thrombosis.

If possible, rinse the wound several times and carefully dispose of the contaminated liquid. Reserve the equipment you used for that particular patient. Dry and store it after soaking it in disinfectant.

Trunk or thigh wounds

Because they're difficult to irrigate, trunk or thigh wounds require some ingenuity. One method uses Stomahesive and a plastic irrigating chamber applied over the wound. (Run warm solution through an infusion set and collect it in a drainage bag.)

You can also use a syringe for irrigation. Where possible, direct the flow at right angles to the wound and allow the fluid to drain by gravity. Doing so requires careful positioning of the patient, either in bed or on a chair. The patient may need analgesia during the treatment.

If irrigation isn't possible, you'll have to swab the wound clean, which is time-consuming. Swab away exudate before using antiseptic or saline solution to clean the wound (taking care not to push loose debris into the wound).

Positioned for success

- Keep the patient positioned to allow further wound drainage into the basin.
- Clean the area around the wound with normal saline solution and pat dry with gauze; wipe intact surrounding skin with a skin protectant wipe and allow it to dry.
- Pack the wound lightly and loosely, if ordered, and apply a dressing.
- Remove and discard your gloves and gown.
- Make sure the patient is comfortable.
- Dispose of drainage, solutions, trash bag, and soiled equipment and supplies according to your facility's policy and Centers for Disease Control and Prevention guidelines.

Practice pointers

- Try to coordinate wound irrigation with the practitioner's or wound care specialist's visit so that he can inspect the wound.
- Irrigate with a bulb syringe if the wound is small or not particularly deep or if a piston syringe is unavailable. However, use a bulb syringe cautiously because this type of syringe doesn't deliver enough pressure to adequately clean the wound.

Debridement

Debridement of nonviable tissue is the most important factor in wound management. Wound healing can't take place until necrotic tissue is removed. Necrotic tissue may present as moist yellow or gray tissue that's separating from viable tissue. If this moist, necrotic tissue becomes dry, it presents as thick, hard, leathery black eschar. Areas of necrotic tissue may mask underlying fluid collections or abscesses. Although debridement can be painful (especially with burns), it's necessary to prevent infection and promote healing of burns and other wounds.

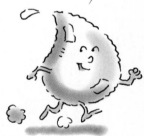

In autolytic debridement, moisture-retentive dressings are placed over the wound and necrotic tissue dissolves in the wound fluid.

Types of debridement

Debridement of necrotic tissue may be accomplished by surgical, autolytic, chemical, or mechanical techniques.

Surgical debridement

Surgical debridement involves removing both necrotic and healthy tissue from the wound bed with a cutting tool. This procedure converts a chronic wound to a clean, acute wound. It's performed only by a doctor in a procedure or operating room with the patient under anesthesia. Caution should be used when performing surgical sharp debridement on patients who have low platelet counts or who are taking anticoagulants.

Autolytic debridement

Autolytic debridement involves the use of moisture-retentive dressings to cover the wound bed. Necrotic tissue is then dissolved through self-digestion of enzymes in the wound fluid. Although autolytic debridement takes longer than other debridement methods, it isn't painful, it's easy to do, and it's appropriate for patients who can't tolerate any other method. Don't perform autolytic debridement if the wound is infected.

Chemical debridement

Chemical debridement with enzymatic agents is a selective method of debridement. Enzymes are applied topically to areas of necrotic tissue only, breaking down necrotic tissue elements. Enzymes digest only necrotic tissue — they don't harm healthy tissue. These agents require specific conditions that vary by product. Effectiveness is achieved by carefully following each manufacturer's guidelines. Stop using the enzymes when the wound is clean with red granulation tissue.

Mechanical debridement

Mechanical debridement includes conservative sharp debridement, wet-to-dry dressings, pulsatile lavage, and hydrotherapy.

Eschar-go

Conservative sharp debridement involves the removal of necrotic tissue only. It's usually performed by a doctor, a physician's assistant, an advanced practice nurse, or certified wound specialist. During conservative sharp debridement, loosened eschar is carefully pryed and cut with forceps and scissors to separate it from viable tissue beneath. One of the most painful types of debridement, it may require either topical or systemic analgesic administration.

Sticky situation

Wet-to-dry dressings, typically used for wounds with extensive necrotic tissue and minimal drainage, require an appropriate technique and the dressing materials used are critical to the outcome. The practitioner places a wet dressing in contact with the lesion and covers it with an outer layer of bandaging. As the dressing dries, it sticks to the wound. When the dried dressing is removed, the necrotic tissue comes off with it.

Finger on the pulse

Pulsatile lavage involves the use of a pressurized antiseptic solution, which cleans tissue and removes wound debris and excess drainage.

Whirlpool wizard

Hydrotherapy — commonly referred to as "tubbing," "tanking," or "whirlpool" — involves immersing the patient in a tank of warm water, with intermittent agitation of the water. It's usually performed on large wounds with a significant amount of nonviable tissue covering the wound surface.

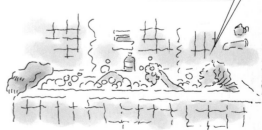

In hydrotherapy, the patient is immersed in a tank of warm water. Now, where's my rubber ducky?

Because you're more likely to be involved in the process of mechanical debridement, these procedures are covered here in detail.

What you need

Ordered pain medication ❋ two pairs of clean or sterile gloves (depending on facility policy) ❋ two gowns or aprons ❋ masks ❋ sterile scissors or sterile scalpel and blade ❋ sterile forceps ❋ sterile 4″ × 4″ gauze pads ❋ appropriate sterile cleaning solutions ❋ sterile marker and labels ❋ sterile dressings ❋ hypoallergenic tape or elastic netting ❋ hemostatic agent, as ordered ❋ needle holder and gut suture with needle (to control bleeding)

How you do it

• Confirm the patient's identity using two patient identifiers according to your facility's policy.
• Provide privacy and explain the procedure to the patient to allay his fears and promote cooperation. Teach him distraction and relaxation techniques, if possible, to minimize his discomfort.
• As ordered, administer an analgesic 20 minutes before debridement begins or give an I.V. analgesic immediately before the procedure.

Conservative sharp debridement

• Keep the patient warm. Expose only the area to be debrided to prevent chilling and fluid and electrolyte loss.
• Wash your hands and then put on clean gloves.
• Remove the wound dressings and clean the wound.
• Remove your dirty gloves and then rewash your hands.
• Set up a sterile field and label all medications, containers, and other solutions on and off the sterile field.
• Help the practitioner put on a gown, mask, and sterile gloves and then put them on yourself.
• Assist the practitioner as he lifts loosened edges of eschar with sterile forceps, holds the necrotic tissue taut with the forceps, and cuts the dead tissue from the wound with the scissors or scalpel blade.
• During the procedure, irrigate the wound as needed.

Slim to none

• Because debridement removes only dead tissue, bleeding should be minimal. If bleeding occurs, apply gentle pressure on

the wound with sterile 4″ × 4″ gauze pads. Then apply the hemo-static agent. If bleeding persists, notify the practitioner and main-tain pressure on the wound. Excessive bleeding or spurting vessels may warrant ligation.
• Perform additional procedures, such as application of topical medications and dressing replacements, as ordered.
• Discard all sharps in a sharps container.

Wet-to-dry dressings

• Put on clean gloves.
• Slowly and gently remove the old dressing, using saline solution to moisten portions of the dressing that don't easily pull away. Discard the old dressing and gloves in a waterproof trash bag.
• Put on sterile gloves.
• Using sterile technique, moisten an open-weave cotton gauze dressing with saline solution and loosely pack it into the wound. Make sure the entire wound surface is lightly covered with moistened gauze.
• Apply an outer dressing and secure it with tape or an adhesive bandage.
• Remove the dressing after it completely dries and becomes adherent to the necrotic tissue (typically in 4 to 6 hours).

Pulsatile lavage

• Use sterile technique to instill a slow, steady stream of sterile normal saline solution into the wound with an irrigating syringe or catheter and concurrently aspirate the solution through a separate suction tube.
• Dry the wound with sterile 4″ × 4″ gauze pads.

Hydrotherapy

• Prepare the tub and obtain the patient's vital signs.
• Help the patient into the tub.
• After the patient or the affected limb has been immersed in the swirling water for the prescribed amount of time (10 to 20 minutes), put on clean gloves, remove the old dressings, and discard all items in a waterproof trash bag.
• Spray rinse and pat dry the patient before reapplying and securing sterile dressings.

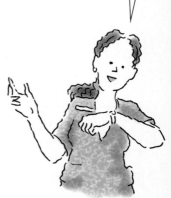

Try to limit debridement to 20 minutes because the procedures are painful.

Practice pointers

• Acknowledge the patient's discomfort and provide pain control and emotional support.

• Work quickly — with an assistant if possible — to complete debridement as fast as possible. Try to limit procedure time to 20 minutes. Serial debridement may be necessary to rid the wound of necrotic tissue.

Wound specimen collection

Wound specimen collection involves using a sterile cotton-tipped swab, aspiration with a syringe, or punch tissue biopsy to help identify pathogens.

Because most wounds are colonized with surface bacteria, the swab specimen technique is limited in that it only obtains surface cultures. Needle aspiration of fluid or punch tissue biopsy is recommended for accurate wound culturing. These techniques are performed by doctors, physician's assistants, advanced practice nurses, or certified wound specialists.

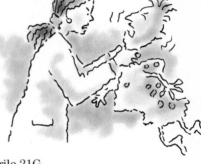

Avoiding contamination with skin bacteria is a key part of wound specimen collection.

What you need

Clean and sterile gloves ❖ alcohol pads or povidone-iodine pads ❖ sterile swabs ❖ sterile 10-ml syringe ❖ sterile 21G needle ❖ sterile culture tube with transport medium (or commercial collection kit for aerobic culture) ❖ labels ❖ special anaerobic culture tube containing carbon dioxide or nitrogen ❖ fresh sterile dressings for the wound ❖ laboratory request form ❖ patient labels

How you do it

• Confirm the patient's identity using two patient identifiers according to your facility's policy.
• Provide privacy and explain the procedure to the patient.
• Wash your hands, prepare a sterile field, and put on clean or sterile gloves.
• Remove the dressing to expose the wound. Dispose of the soiled dressings properly.
• Put on a new pair of gloves.
• Clean the wound well.
• Inspect the wound, noting the color, amount, and odor of drainage and the presence of necrotic debris.
• Clean the area around the wound with an alcohol pad or a povidone-iodine pad to reduce the risk of contaminating the speci-

men with skin bacteria. Then allow the area to dry. Remember to make sure that antiseptic doesn't enter the wound.

Aerobic culture

- Compress the edges of the wound to elicit new drainage.
- Rotate a sterile cotton-tipped swab on the sides and base of the wound bed. If the wound is dry, dip the swab into the transport medium to moisten the tip before swabbing the base of the wound. Remember, never collect exudate from the skin and then insert the same swab into the wound; this could contaminate the wound with skin bacteria.
- Remove the swab from the wound and immediately place it in the aerobic culture tube.
- Label the culture tube and send the tube to the laboratory immediately with a completed laboratory request form. Remember to note antibiotic therapy on the request form.

Anaerobic culture

- Obtain a wound fluid sample as described. Immediately place it in the anaerobic culture tube (see *Anaerobic specimen collector*).
- Or, insert a sterile 10-ml syringe, without a needle, into the wound and aspirate 1 to 5 ml of exudate into the syringe. Then attach the 21G needle to the syringe and immediately inject the aspirate into the anaerobic culture tube.
- Label the culture tube and send it to the laboratory immediately with a completed laboratory request form. Remember to note antibiotic therapy on the request form.
- If an anaerobic culture tube is unavailable, obtain a rubber stopper, attach the needle to the syringe, and gently push all the air out of the syringe by pressing on the plunger. Stick the needle tip into the rubber stopper, remove and discard your gloves, and send the syringe of aspirate to the laboratory immediately with a completed laboratory request form.

Practice pointers

- Although you would normally clean the area around a wound to prevent contamination by normal skin flora, don't clean a perineal wound with alcohol because this could irritate sensitive tissues.
- If rotating the swab in the wound doesn't provide a specimen, try using a Z-stroke (zig-zag) motion over the entire wound bed.

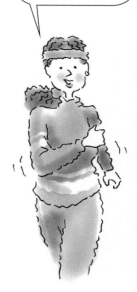

I love doing aerobics! Oh, we're talking about aerobic and anaerobic cultures? In that case, remember to label your culture tubes.

Anaerobic specimen collector

Because most anaerobes die when exposed to oxygen, they must be transported in tubes filled with carbon dioxide or nitrogen. The anaerobic specimen collector shown here includes a tube filled with carbon dioxide, a small inner tube, and a swab attached to a plastic plunger.

   Before specimen collection, the small inner tube containing the swab is held in place with the rubber stopper (as shown below left). After collecting the specimen, quickly replace the swab in the inner tube and depress the plunger to separate the inner tube from the stopper (as shown below right), forcing it into the larger tube and exposing the specimen to a carbon dioxide-rich environment.

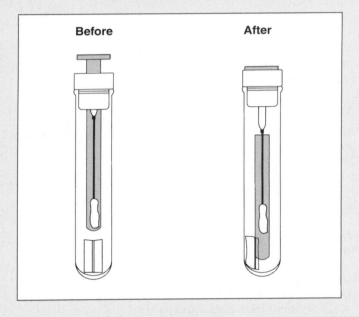

Before   **After**

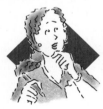

Quick quiz

1. Because mechanical debridement is painful, the procedure should be limited to:

    A.   5 minutes.
    B.   10 minutes.
    C.   20 minutes.
    D.   25 minutes.

Answer: C. Debridement should be performed for no more than 20 minutes. If needed, the procedure can be repeated to completely remove the necrotic tissue.

2. To irrigate a wound, direct the flow of irrigant:
  A. toward the wound.
  B. away from the wound.
  C. toward the center of the wound.
  D. to pool inside of the wound.

Answer: B. Direct the flow away from the wound to prevent contamination.

3. The most commonly used cleaning agent is:
  A. normal saline solution.
  B. hydrogen peroxide.
  C. povidone-iodine solution.
  D. sodium hypochlorite.

Answer: A. Sterile normal saline solution is most commonly used because it provides a moist environment, promotes granulation tissue formation, and causes minimal fluid shifts in healthy adults.

4. Which type of dressing wouldn't be appropriate for a wound with excessive drainage?
  A. Gauze dressing
  B. Transparent film dressing
  C. Alginate dressing
  D. Hydrocolloid dressing

Answer: B. Because a transparent film dressing can't absorb drainage, it should be used only for wounds with minimal drainage.

5. Which methods of wound culturing are most accurate for determining infection?
  A. Swab technique and needle aspiration
  B. Swab technique and punch tissue biopsy
  C. Needle aspiration and punch tissue biopsy
  D. Aerobic and anaerobic swab techniques

Answer: C. Because the surface of most wounds is normally colonized with bacteria, swab cultures may not be accurate. Needle aspiration and punch tissue biopsy provide the most reliable information.

Scoring

☆☆☆ If you answered all five questions correctly, yippee! You're quite a fine specimen.

☆☆ If you answered four questions correctly, great job! You really cleaned up in the area of basic wound care procedures.

☆ If you answered fewer than four questions correctly, don't despair! Irrigate your system and then review the chapter again.

Acute wounds

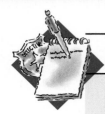

Just the facts

In this chapter, you'll learn:

♦ types of acute wounds, including those caused by surgery, trauma, and burns

♦ assessment factors for each type of acute wound

♦ ways in which skin grafts are used to repair defects caused by acute wounds.

A look at acute wounds

Three criteria are generally used to classify wounds and determine their severity: age, depth, and color. However, to determine a wound's age, you must first determine if it's acute or chronic. To do this, you shouldn't adhere solely to a timeline; you should also consider the wound's progress toward healing. Ask these questions when characterizing an acute wound:

• Is the wound new or relatively new?

• Did the wound occur suddenly (as opposed to developing over time)?

• Is the wound healing in a timely, predictable, and measurable manner?

Intent or accident?

Acute wounds can occur by intention or trauma. For example, a surgical incision is an acute wound that's caused intentionally. Traumatic wounds can range from simple to severe. Burns are a category of traumatic wound that have a unique set of causes, potential complications, and treatment options.

Regardless of the cause, when caring for a patient with an acute wound, you'll focus on restoring normal anatomic structure, physiologic function, and appearance to the wound area (sometimes accomplished by skin grafting).

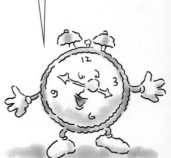

Time isn't the only distinguishing factor when determining whether a wound is acute or chronic.

Surgical wounds

An acute surgical wound is a healthy and uncomplicated break in the skin's continuity resulting from surgery. In an otherwise healthy individual, this type of wound responds well to postoperative care and heals without incident in a predictable period of time.

Factors that affect healing

Several factors can greatly affect the course of postoperative wound healing. These include the patient's age, nutritional status, general health before surgery, and oxygenation status.

Age

Age is an important factor in the healing process, especially for pediatric patients and older adults. Premature infants and infants up to age 1 have immature immune systems and are therefore at greater risk for infection before, during, and after surgery. At the other end of the age continuum, older adults commonly have a harder time healing after surgery due to skin changes. As a person ages, skin becomes thinner and less elastic. (See *Age and wound healing*.)

Nutrition

Proper nutrition is crucial for the body to heal itself effectively. During your assessment, it's imperative for you to identify nutritional problems early and to develop a plan that addresses deficits.

After surgery, the body quickly depletes its stores of nutrients (especially in the highly exudative wound) and even an otherwise healthy patient can become malnourished if diet is ignored. The care plan must include a diet with adequate nutrients to maintain homeostasis and create an optimum environment for wound healing.

Adipose poses problems

A patient who's overweight has an additional problem. Adipose tissue lacks the extensive vascular supply present in skin. As the amount of adipose tissue increases, blood flow to the skin decreases. This reduces the amount of oxygen and nutrients reaching the wound area, which impedes healing and increases the risk of wound dehiscence.

Because the body quickly depletes its nutrient stores after surgery, be sure to include a balanced diet with adequate nutrients in your care plan.

Handle with care

Age and wound healing

In infants and elderly patients, surgical wounds may not heal normally.

Infants

In premature infants and infants up to age 1, the immune system and other body systems aren't fully developed, so there's a greater risk for infection before, during, and after surgery. Sterile technique is a critical component of care for very young patients.

Elderly patients

Skin becomes thinner and less elastic with age. Populations of cells that repair tissues and fight infection decline and the skin's vascular system is less robust. As a result, surgical wounds in elderly patients heal more slowly, increasing the risk of infection.

Illness or infection

In most cases, a preexisting illness or infection delays or complicates healing after surgery. Unfortunately, it isn't always possible to delay surgery while an underlying condition resolves itself. In these cases, the care plan must include measures that minimize the impact of the preexisting condition on the healing process. For example:

• Disorders that impede blood flow, such as coronary artery disease, peripheral vascular disease (PVD), and hypertension, can cause problems by reducing the flow of blood reaching the incision site. A patient with one of these conditions requires a care plan that includes interventions to improve circulation.

• Cancer may necessitate more aggressive pain management or a care plan that includes management of such symptoms as nausea and vomiting.

• Diabetes mellitus impedes healing in many ways and increases the patient's risk of infection. Diabetic neuropathy (inflammation and degeneration of peripheral nerves), if present, may interfere with vasodilation and, consequently, circulation in the area of the incision.

• Immunosuppression resulting from either a disease or drug therapy (corticosteroids, chemotherapy) may impair the inflammatory response, delaying wound healing and increasing the patient's risk of infection.

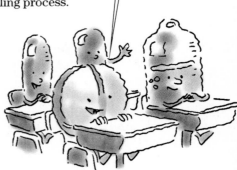

Did you hear that? Some drugs cause immunosuppression, which delays wound healing and increases the risk of infection.

Stopping on red

A preexisting infection can also delay or impair healing. Signs of wound infection include:
- increased exudate
- purulent (pus-containing) exudate
- erythema (reddened tissue) around the wound
- warmer skin temperature at or around the wound
- new or increased pain
- general malaise
- fever
- high white blood cell (WBC) count.

All open wounds are colonized with surface bacteria but infected wounds are slow to heal and may become dehisced or eviscerated.

Oxygenation status

During healing, neutrophils require oxygen to produce the hydrogen peroxide they use to kill pathogens, and fibroblasts require oxygen for collagen proliferation. Therefore, adequate oxygenation is critical to the healing process. Any condition that impedes overall oxygenation or the amount of oxygen reaching the wound—atherosclerosis, for example—slows the healing process.

Assessment and care

Your care should focus on keeping the wound clean and protecting it from trauma. Proper care during healing varies depending on the method of wound closure used, the development of the healing ridge, and the type of dressing ordered. The patient's ability to properly perform wound care after discharge also affects healing.

Wound closure

The surgeon determines the appropriate method of wound closure based on the wound's severity; in most cases, sutures are used.

Sew...a needle pulling thread

In suturing, a natural or synthetic thread is used to stitch the wound closed. (See *Suture materials and methods*.)

Sutures typically remain in place for 7 to 10 days, depending on the wound's severity, the type of tissue involved, and whether healing is progressing as expected. Factors that affect the timing of suture removal include the patient's overall condition; the

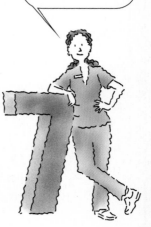

Sutures typically remain in place for 7 to 10 days, as long as no complications are present.

Suture materials and methods

When closing a surgical wound, the choice of suture material varies according to the suturing method, location, and tissue type.

Materials

Nonabsorbable sutures:
- are used to close the skin surface
- provide strength and immobility
- cause minimal tissue irritation
- are made of silk, cotton, stainless steel, or Dacron.

   Absorbable sutures:
- are used when suture removal is undesirable (for example, sutures in an underlying tissue layer)
- are made of chromic catgut (a natural catgut treated with chromium trioxide to improve strength and prolong absorption time), plain catgut (a material that's absorbed faster and is more likely to cause irritation than chromic catgut), or synthetic materials (such as polyglycolic acid) that are replacing catgut because they're stronger, more durable, and less irritating.

Methods

The most common suture methods include mattress continuous suture, plain continuous suture, mattress interrupted suture, plain interrupted suture, and blanket continuous suture.

Mattress continuous suture

Connected mattress stitches with a knot at the beginning and end.

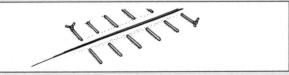

Plain continuous suture

Connected stitches with the thread knotted at the beginning and end of the suture (also called a *continuous running suture*).

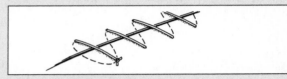

Mattress interrupted suture

Independent stitches with both threads crossing beneath the suture line, leaving only a small portion of suture exposed on each side of the wound.

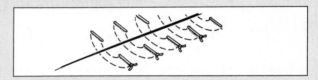

Plain interrupted suture

Individual sutures sewn with a separate piece of thread. Half the thread length crosses under the suture line and the other half crosses above the skin surface.

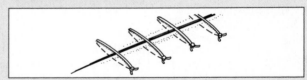

Blanket continuous suture

Looped stitches with a knot at the beginning and end.

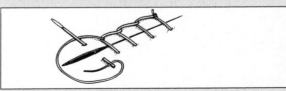

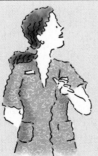

shape, size, and location of the incision; and whether inflammation, drainage, or infection develops.

Stainless steel solutions

The surgeon may choose to use skin staples or clips as an alternative to sutures if cosmetic results aren't an issue. These closures secure a wound faster than sutures and, because they're made of surgical stainless steel, tissue reaction is minimal. Properly placed staples and clips distribute tension evenly along the suture line, reducing tissue trauma and compression. This promotes healing and minimizes scarring. The surgeon won't use staples or clips if less than 5 mm of tissue exists between the staple and any underlying bone, vessel, or organ. (See *Using retention sutures.*)

Stick with me!

Smaller wounds with little drainage can be closed with adhesive skin closures, such as Steri-Strips or butterfly closures. As with staples and clips, these closures cause little tissue reaction. Adhesive closures can be used after suture or staple removal to provide ongoing support for a healing incision. (See *Types of adhesive skin closures.*)

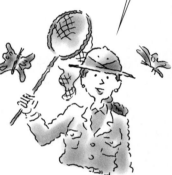

Butterfly closures can be used to promote healing after suture removal.

The healing ridge

To properly assess healing, it's important to understand how the healing ridge develops in an incision after surgery. The healing ridge is a buildup of collagen fibers that begins to form during the inflammatory phase of wound healing (usually the first 24 to 72 hours) and peaks during the proliferation phase (usually between days 5 and 9). You should feel this ridge as you gently palpate the skin on each side of the wound. The healing ridge is a sign that healing is progressing. If you can't feel the ridge, healing isn't progressing as expected, further assessment is required, and you

---

Handle with care

Using retention sutures

Although not used exclusively for bariatric patients, retention sutures can be used to secure wound edges and to support the suture line. The use of retention sutures for bariatric patients helps support the deep tissues while the more superficial fascia and skin tissues heal. Retention sutures are placed through the abdominal wall before the abdominal layers are closed to reinforce the suture line.

Types of adhesive skin closures

The two most common types of adhesive skin closures are Steri-Strips and butterfly closures.

Steri-Strips
Steri-Strips (thin strips of sterile, nonwoven tape) are a primary means of holding a wound closed after suture removal.

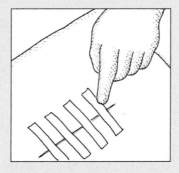

Butterfly closures
Butterfly closures have two sterile, waterproof adhesive strips linked by a narrow, nonadhesive "bridge." They're used to hold small wounds closed to promote healing after suture removal.

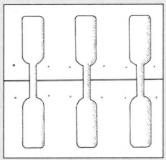

should notify the practitioner. In cases where the ridge fails to develop, mechanical strain on the wound is most likely at fault.

Dressings
The incision dressing shields the wound against pathogens and protects the skin surface from irritating drainage. The dressing is the primary aspect of wound management for surgical wounds; therefore, choosing the right type is important.

Proper dress required
Typically, lightly exuding wounds with drains and wounds with minimal purulent drainage require only loose packing and a gauze cover dressing. A wound with copious, excoriating drainage requires an absorbent dressing, such as an alginate, or pouching to contain the drainage and protect the surrounding skin. (See *Pouching a wound*, page 78.)

Get wise to wounds

Pouching a wound

If your patient's wound is draining heavily or if drainage may damage surrounding skin, you need to apply a pouch. Here's how:
• Measure the wound. Cut an opening ⅜" larger than the wound in the facing of the collection pouch (see photo below).

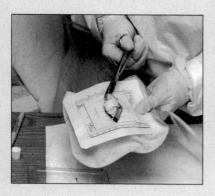

• Apply a skin protectant as needed. (Some protectants are incorporated into the collection pouch system and also provide adhesion.)

• Be sure to close the drainage port at the bottom of the pouch to prevent leaks. Then gently press the contoured pouch opening around the wound, starting at the lower edge, to catch any drainage (see photo below).

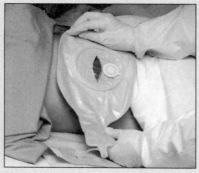

• To empty the pouch, put on gloves, a face shield or mask, and eye protection. Insert the lower portion of the pouch into a graduated biohazard container and open the drainage port (see photo top right). Note the color, consistency, odor, and amount of fluid. If ordered, obtain a culture specimen and send it to

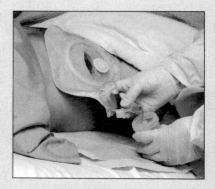

the laboratory immediately. (Always follow the Centers for Disease Control and Prevention's standard precautions when handling infectious drainage.)
• Use a gauze pad to wipe the bottom of the pouch and the drainage port. This prevents skin irritation or possible odor from any residual drainage. Reseal the port.
• Change the pouch only if it leaks or fails to adhere. More frequent changes are unnecessary and can irritate the patient's skin.

When dressing a surgical wound, use sterile technique and sterile supplies to prevent contamination. Change the dressing as often as needed to absorb drainage and keep the surrounding skin dry; however, remember that a wound heals best at body temperature. Changing the dressing lowers the temperature at the wound site, which slows healing until the site returns to normal body temperature.

Teaching about surgical wound care

Surgical patients need to know the ways that they can promote healing and prevent infection. Be sure to discuss:
• signs and symptoms of wound infection to report to the practitioner immediately, such as increased tenderness, deep or increased pain at the wound site, fever, or edema (especially if it occurs between postoperative days 3 and 5)
• how to take an accurate temperature reading
• proper wound care, such as the importance of keeping the incision clean and dry; proper hand-washing technique; and the supplies and methods used to clean the wound
• wound dressings, including the type, where to obtain them, and how to apply them
• types and levels of permissible activity, such as lifting restrictions (if applicable), when the patient may shower or bathe, and when he can expect to return to work
• follow-up appointments.

Patient education

Patient education is an important component of the care plan for patients with surgical wounds. By the time he's discharged, the patient needs to understand — and demonstrate — the ability to perform proper wound care. Start with an assessment of the patient's knowledge. Then begin your teaching with a discussion of basic asepsis and hand-washing techniques. The balance of your teaching depends on the type of surgery, the type of dressing, and the location of the wound. (See *Teaching about surgical wound care.*)

Potential complications

Surgery results in a controlled form of acute wound. The patient's environment, the type and severity of the wound, and preoperative and postoperative care are all under the control of the health care team. Consequently, most surgical wounds heal without incident; however, some complications that might arise include infection, hemorrhage, and dehiscence and evisceration.

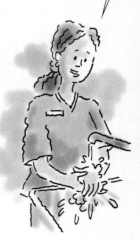

Start patient teaching with the basics — asepsis and hand-washing techniques.

Handle with care

Acute wound complications in bariatric patients

Bariatric patients are at an increased risk for acute wound complications, including infection, dehiscence caused by increased tension on wound edges at the time of wound closure, and hematoma formation caused by pooled blood.

These complications may be the result of many factors, including:
- difficulty level of operating on these patients
- lengthier operation time, which increases the chances of contamination
- increased trauma (for example, the more forceful retraction needed during surgery may cause necrosis of the abdominal wall).

Infection

Wound infection is the most common wound complication as well as the second most common health care–associated infection. Preventing wound infection requires meticulous attention to sterile technique when caring for an acute wound. (See *Acute wound complications in bariatric patients.*)

Mean to intervene

For a surgical patient, wound infection is a significant and serious event requiring prompt intervention. Interventions typically ordered in cases of postoperative infection include:
- obtaining a wound culture and sensitivity test
- administering antibiotics
- irrigating the wound
- dressing the wound and loosely packing it, if necessary
- monitoring wound drainage.

Hemorrhage

Hemorrhage may occur from damage to blood vessels. In the postoperative patient, it may happen in either internal or external sites. The most common locations of significant internal hemorrhages are:
- posterior nasal passages
- pulmonary vessels
- spleen
- liver
- stomach
- uterus.

Hemorrhage may also occur at the site of a large artery injury or aneurysm. Hemorrhage in one of these

I'm one of the most common locations of postoperative internal hemorrhage. Yikes!

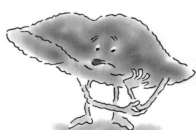

areas significantly reduces the volume of circulating blood and precipitates hypovolemia. Nursing interventions include administering I.V. fluids to increase blood pressure and urine output and determining the source of bleeding. If the hemorrhage originates externally—for example, from the wound itself or from damage to the fragile, newly developed blood vessels—place pressure or a pressure dressing on the site of the bleeding and notify the practitioner for specific treatment orders.

Dehiscence and evisceration

Dehiscence is most likely to occur when collagen fibers aren't mature enough to hold the incision closed without sutures. The first sign of dehiscence may be an abscess or a gush of serosanguineous fluid from the wound or a report from the patient of a "popping" sensation after sneezing, coughing, or retching. Complete dehiscence leads to evisceration, in which underlying tissues protrude through the wound opening. Abdominal wounds are more likely to dehisce and eviscerate than thoracic wounds.

An ounce of prevention

To prevent wound dehiscence and evisceration, teach the patient to support the incision with a pillow or cushion before he changes position, coughs, or sneezes.

If dehiscence occurs, take these steps:
• Stay with the patient; keep him still and have a colleague notify the practitioner.
• If the patient has an abdominal wound, help him into low Fowler's position, with his knees bent to reduce abdominal tension.
• If evisceration is evident, cover extruding tissues with abdominal dressings saturated with sterile normal saline solution.

Traumatic wounds

A traumatic wound is a sudden, unplanned injury to the skin that can range from minor (such as a skinned knee) to severe (such as a gunshot wound).

Types of traumatic wounds

Traumatic wounds include abrasions, lacerations, skin tears, bites, and penetrating trauma wounds.

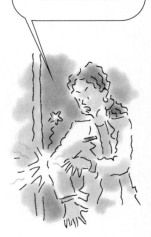

Ouch! It may not seem too traumatic, but even a minor abrasion such as a skinned elbow is considered a traumatic wound.

Abrasions

An abrasion occurs when a mechanical force, such as friction or shearing, scrapes away a partial thickness of the skin. Unless an unusually large amount of skin is involved or an infection develops, an abrasion is one of the least complicated traumatic wounds.

Lacerations

A laceration is a tear in the skin that's caused by a sharp object, such as metal, glass, or wood. It can also be caused by trauma that produces high shearing force. A laceration has jagged, irregular edges and its severity depends on its cause, size, depth, and location.

Skin tears

A skin tear is a specific type of laceration that most often affects older adults. In a skin tear, friction alone — or shearing force plus friction — separates layers of skin. A partial-thickness wound occurs if the epidermis separates from the dermis; a full-thickness wound occurs if the epidermis and dermis separate from underlying tissue. Use a classification system, such as Payne-Martin, to classify skin tears during assessment. (See *Classifying skin tears*.) This type of injury may be preventable through careful handling by members of the health care team. (See *Preventing skin tears*.)

Bites

When assessing a bite wound, it's important to quickly discover the bite's source — cat, dog, bat, snake, spider, human? This helps the health care team determine which bacteria or toxins may be present and the likely type of tissue trauma.

Hannibal the cannibal?

For example, a human bite can cause a puncture wound and introduce any one of the innumerable organisms present in the human mouth into the wound. *Staphylococcus aureus* and streptococci are two such organisms that can be transmitted to the wound or into the victim's bloodstream. Other serious diseases that can be transmitted in this way include human immunodeficiency virus infection, hepatitis B, hepatitis C, syphilis, and tuberculosis. Some evidence suggests that a human bite can also cause necrotizing fasciitis (rapidly progressing skin infection usually caused by two types of organisms).

Animal house

A bite from a dog, cat, or rodent can introduce deadly infectious diseases, such as rabies, into a wound. Cats and

---

Classifying skin tears

To provide consistent assessment of skin tears, utilize a classification system such as the Payne-Martin system to document your findings.

The Payne-Martin system classifies skin tears as:
• Category I — skin tear without tissue loss
• Category II — skin tear with partial tissue loss
• Category III — skin tear with complete tissue loss, in which the epidermal flap is absent.

Be aware that bites from animals, such as dogs, cats, and rabbits, can cause rabies in addition to possible tissue damage.

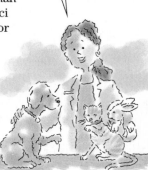

Preventing skin tears

As aging occurs, the skin becomes more prone to skin tear injuries. Prevent skin tears by using:
• proper lifting, positioning, transferring, and turning techniques to reduce or eliminate friction or shear
• padding on support surfaces where the risk is greatest, such as bed rails and limb supports on a wheelchair, and over skin when limb restraints are used
• pillows or cushions to support the patient's arms and legs
• nonadhering dressings or those with minimal adherent such as paper tape
• a skin barrier wipe before applying dressings
• the push-pull technique to cautiously remove tape or other adhesives
• wraps, such as a stockinette or soft gauze, to protect areas of skin where the risk of tearing is high
• skin lotion applied twice per day to areas at risk.
    Be sure to tell your patient to:
• add protection by wearing long-sleeved shirts and long pants, as weather permits
• avoid sudden or brusque movements that can pull the skin and possibly cause a skin tear.

other smaller mammals cause relatively little tissue damage. However, a dog can generate up to 200 psi of pressure when biting and if he shakes his head at the same time (which is usually the case), strong torsional force is brought to bear. Together, these forces can cause a massive amount of tissue damage.

Penetrating trauma wounds

A penetrating trauma wound is a puncture wound. This type of wound may be the result of an accident or a personal attack, as in the case of a stabbing or gunshot wound.

Knife strife

A stab wound is a low-velocity wound that generally presents as a classic puncture wound or laceration. In some cases, it may involve organ damage beneath the wound site. X-rays, computed tomography scanning, and magnetic resonance imaging are used to evaluate possible organ damage. If the weapon used was contaminated, the patient is at risk for local infection, sepsis, and tetanus.

Smoking gun

A gunshot wound is a high-velocity wound. Factors that affect the severity of tissue damage include the caliber of the weapon, the velocity of the projectile, and the patient's position at the time of injury.

In most cases, a small-caliber weapon firing a relatively low-velocity projectile creates a small, clean punctuate lesion with little or no bleeding. If the projectile is no longer in the patient's body, treat this lesion as you would any other open wound.

A large-caliber, relatively high-velocity projectile typically causes massive tissue destruction, a large gaping wound, profuse bleeding, and wound contamination. In this case, the patient usually requires immediate surgical intervention. After surgery, treat the wound as a surgical wound.

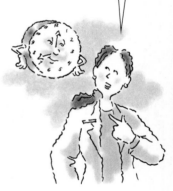

Time is critical when caring for a patient with a traumatic wound.

Assessment and care

Time is critical when caring for a patient with a traumatic wound. First, assess airway, breathing, and circulation (ABCs). Although focusing first on the injury itself may seem natural, a patent airway and pumping heart take priority.

Next, turn your attention to the wound. Control bleeding by applying firm, direct pressure and elevate the patient's extremities. If bleeding continues, you may need to compress a pressure point above the wound. Then assess the wound's condition. Specific wound management and cleaning depend on the type of wound and degree of contamination. (See *Caring for a patient with a traumatic wound.*)

Special considerations

When caring for a patient with a traumatic wound, pay particular attention to these aspects of care:
• Avoid using more than 8 psi of pressure when irrigating the wound. High-pressure irrigation can seriously interfere with healing by destroying cells and forcing bacteria into the tissue.
• Use sterile normal saline solution to remove debris when cleaning the wound. Never instill hydrogen peroxide into a deep wound because the evolving gases can cause an embolism.
• Avoid using alcohol to clean a traumatic wound. It's painful for the patient and dehydrates tissue. Similarly, avoid cleaning with antiseptics because they can impede healing.
• Never use a cotton ball or a cotton-filled gauze pad to clean a wound because cotton fibers left in the wound may cause contamination or a foreign body reaction.

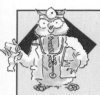

Get wise to wounds

Caring for a patient with a traumatic wound

When treating a patient with a traumatic wound, always begin by assessing the ABCs: airway, breathing, and circulation. Move on to the wound itself only after ABCs are stable. Here are the basic steps to follow when caring for each type of traumatic wound.

Abrasion
• Flush the area of the abrasion with normal saline solution or wound cleaning solution.
• Use a sterile 4″ × 4″ gauze pad moistened with normal saline solution to remove dirt or gravel and gently rub toward the entry point to work contaminants back out the way they entered.
• If the wound is extremely dirty, it may need to be scrubbed with a surgical brush. This should be ordered and supervised by a practitioner. Be as gentle as possible and keep in mind that this is a painful process for your patient.
• Allow a small wound to dry and form a scab. Cover larger wounds with a nonadherent pad or petroleum gauze and a light dressing. Apply antibacterial ointment if ordered.

Laceration
• Moisten a sterile 4″ × 4″ gauze pad with normal saline solution or wound cleaning solution. Gently clean the wound, beginning at the center and working out to about 2″ (5 cm) beyond the edge of the wound. Whenever the pad becomes soiled, discard it and use a new one. Continue until the wound appears clean.
• If necessary, irrigate the wound using a 50-ml catheter-tip syringe and normal saline solution.
• Assist the practitioner in suturing the wound if necessary; apply sterile strips of porous tape if suturing isn't needed.
• Apply antibacterial ointment as ordered to prevent infection.

• Apply a dry sterile dressing over the wound to absorb drainage and help prevent bacterial contamination.

Bite
• Immediately irrigate the wound with copious amounts of normal saline solution. Don't immerse and soak the wound because this may allow bacteria to float back into the tissue.
• Clean the wound with sterile 4″ × 4″ gauze pads and an antiseptic solution such as povidone-iodine.
• Assist with debridement, if ordered.
• Apply a loose dressing. If the bite is on an extremity, elevate it to reduce swelling.
• Ask the patient about the animal that bit him to determine whether there's a risk of rabies. Administer rabies and tetanus shots, as needed.

Penetrating wound
• If the wound is minor, allow it to bleed for a few minutes before cleaning it. A larger puncture wound may require irrigation.
• Cover the wound with a dry dressing.
• If the wound contains an embedded foreign object, such as a shard of glass or metal, stabilize the object until the practitioner can remove it. When the object is removed and bleeding is under control, clean the wound as you would a laceration.
• Administer tetanus vaccine, as needed.

• If the practitioner plans to debride the wound to remove dead tissue and reduce the risk of infection and scarring, loosely pack the wound with gauze pads soaked in normal saline solution until it's time for the procedure.
• Monitor closely for signs of developing infection, such as warm red skin or purulent discharge from the wound. Infection in a traumatic wound can delay healing, increase scarring, and trigger systemic infections such as septicemia.
• Inspect the dressing regularly. If edema develops, adjust the dressing to ensure adequate circulation to the affected area of the wound.

Burns

The degree of tissue damage caused by a burn depends on the strength of the source and the duration of contact or exposure.

Types of burns

A burn is an acute wound caused by exposure to thermal extremes, electricity, caustic chemicals, or radiation.

Thermal burns

The most common type of burn, thermal burns can result from virtually any misuse or mishandling of fire or a combustible product. Playing with matches, pouring gasoline into a hot lawnmower, and setting off fireworks are some common examples of ways in which burns occur. Thermal burns can also result from kitchen accidents, house or office fires, automobile accidents, or physical abuse. Although it's less common, exposure to extreme cold can also cause thermal burns.

Electrical burns

Electrical burns result from contact with flowing electrical current. Household current, high-voltage transmission lines, and lightning are sources of electrical burns.

Chemical burns

Chemical burns most commonly result from contact (skin contact or inhalation) with a caustic agent, such as an acid, an alkali, or a vesicant.

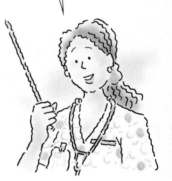

Types of burns include thermal, electrical, chemical, and radiation burns.

Radiation burns

The most common radiation burn is sunburn, which follows excessive exposure to the sun. Almost all other burns due to radiation exposure occur as a result of radiation treatment or in specific industries that use or process radioactive materials.

Factors that affect healing

Factors that affect treatment and healing include:
• burn location — burns on the face, hands, feet, and genitalia are most serious due to the possible loss of function
• burn configuration — edema due to a circumferential burn (completely encircling an extremity) can slow or stop circulation

to the extremity; burns on the neck can obstruct the airway; burns on the chest can interfere with normal respiration by inhibiting expansion
• preexisting medical conditions—note disorders that impair peripheral circulation, especially diabetes, PVD, and chronic alcohol abuse
• other injuries sustained at the time of the burn
• patient age—patients younger than age 4 or older than age 60 are at higher risk for complications and, consequently, for a higher mortality rate
• pulmonary injury—inhaling smoke or super-heated air damages lung tissue.

Assessment

Conduct your initial assessment as soon as possible after the burn occurs. First, assess the patient's ABCs. Then determine the patient's level of consciousness and mobility. Next, assess the burn, including its size, depth, and severity.

Determining size

Determine burn size as part of your initial assessment. Typically, burn size is expressed as a percentage of total body surface area (BSA). The Rule of Nines and the Lund-Browder Classification are two useful tools for providing reasonably standardized and quick estimates of the percentage of BSA affected. (See *Estimating burn size*, page 88.)

Determining depth

During the initial assessment, determine the depth of tissue damage. A partial-thickness burn damages the epidermis and part of the dermis. A full-thickness burn involves the epidermis, dermis, and subcutaneous tissue.

Four degrees of separation

The traditional method of gauging burn severity classified burn depth by degree. Today, most assessment findings use depth of tissue damage to describe a burn:
• Superficial partial-thickness (first-degree)—damage is limited to the epidermis, causing erythema and pain
• Deep partial-thickness (second-degree)—the epidermis and part of the dermis are damaged, producing blisters, mild-to-moderate edema, and pain
• Full-thickness (third-degree)—the epidermis and dermis are damaged with damage extending into the subcutaneous tissue layer; may also involve muscle, bone, and interstitial tissues.

Memory jogger

To remember the proper sequence for the initial assessment of a burn patient, remember your ABCs and add D and E.

Airway — Assess the patient's airway, remove any obstruction, and treat any obstructive condition.

Breathing — Observe the motion of the patient's chest. Auscultate the depth, rate, and characteristics of the patient's breathing.

Circulation — Palpate the patient's pulse at the carotid artery and then at the distal pulse points in the wrist, posterior tibial area, and foot. Loss of distal pulse may indicate shock or constriction of an extremity.

Disability — Assess the patient's level of consciousness and ability to function before attempting to move or transfer him.

Expose — Remove burned clothing from burned areas of the patient's body and thoroughly examine the skin beneath.

Estimating burn size

Because body surface area (BSA) varies with age, two different methods are used to estimate burn size in adult and pediatric patients.

Rule of Nines

You can quickly estimate the extent of an adult patient's burn by using the Rule of Nines. This method quantifies BSA in multiples of 9, thus the name. To use this method, mentally transfer the burns on your patient to the body charts below. Add the corresponding percentages for each body section burned. Use the total—a rough estimate of burn extent—to calculate initial fluid replacement needs.

Lund-Browder Classification

The Rule of Nines isn't accurate for infants or children because their body shapes, and therefore BSA, differ from those of adults. For example, an infant's head accounts for about 17% of his total BSA, compared with 7% for an adult. Instead, use the Lund-Browder Classification to determine burn size for infants and children.

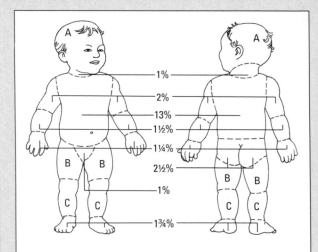

Percentage of burned body surface by age

At birth	0 to 1 year	1 to 4 years	5 to 9 years	10 to 15 years	Adult
A: Half of head					
9½%	8½%	6½%	5½%	4½%	3½%
B: Half of one thigh					
2¾%	3¼%	4%	4¼%	4½%	4¾%
C: Half of one leg					
2½%	2½%	2¾%	3%	3¼%	3½%

Visualizing burn depth

The most widely used system of classifying burn depth and severity categorizes burns by degree. However, it's important to remember that most burns involve tissue damage of different degrees and thicknesses. This illustration may help you visualize burn damage at the various degrees.

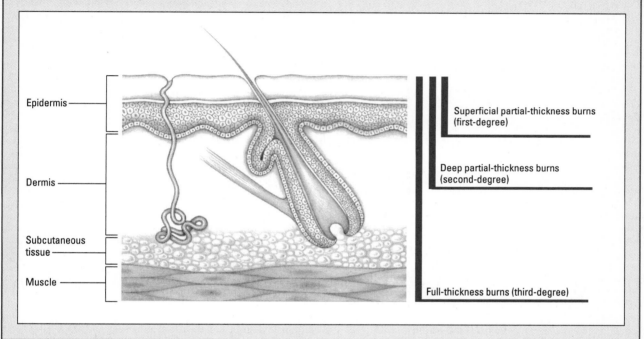

Epidermis

Dermis

Subcutaneous tissue

Muscle

Superficial partial-thickness burns (first-degree)

Deep partial-thickness burns (second-degree)

Full-thickness burns (third-degree)

In most instances, damage involves several depths and degrees. (See *Visualizing burn depth.*)

Determining severity

The severity of a burn is associated with both its size and depth. The three categories of burn severity are major, moderate, and minor.

Major

Major burns meet one or more of these criteria:
• full-thickness burns on more than 10% of BSA
• deep partial-thickness burns on more than 25% of BSA in adults; more than 20% in children
• burns on the hands, face, feet, or genitalia
• burns complicated by fractures or respiratory damage
• electrical burns
• any burn in a high-risk patient.

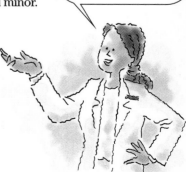

Remember, when determining burn severity, you must consider not only the size of the wound but also its depth.

Moderate

Moderate burns meet one or more of these criteria:
- full-thickness burns on 2% to 10% of BSA
- deep partial-thickness burns on 15% to 25% of BSA in adults, 10% to 20% in children.

Minor

Minor burns meet one or more of these criteria:
- full-thickness burns on less than 2% of BSA
- deep partial-thickness burns on less than 15% of BSA in adults, less than 10% in children.

Burn care

Care for a patient with a burn depends on the type and severity of the burn, the patient's general health before the injury, and whether another injury was sustained concurrent with the burn. In general, treatment seeks to reduce pain; remove dirt, debris, and dead tissue; and provide a dressing that promotes healing. In some cases, treatment includes skin grafting.

Minor to moderate burns

In minor to moderate burns, the first step is to stop the burning process and relieve pain. Remove smoldering clothing and provide pain medication, as ordered. When cleaning the burns, never use hydrogen peroxide or povidone-iodine (or products containing these agents) because they can cause further tissue damage. Cover the burns with dry, sterile towels.

Something to talk about

As soon as the patient's condition stabilizes, and other injuries are ruled out, the practitioner may order an opioid analgesic, such as morphine or meperidine. Be sure to talk to the patient as you work. Emotional support and reassurance are important aspects of care and may reduce the patient's need for analgesia.

Wrapping it up

After the practitioner debrides devitalized tissue, if necessary, cover the wound with an antimicrobial and a non-

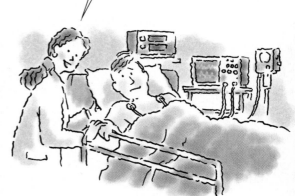

Always talk to your patient while providing burn care. Reassurance may reduce his need for analgesia.

adhesive bulky dressing. If ordered, administer tetanus prophylaxis.

Moderate to major burns

In moderate to major burns, immediately assess the patient's ABCs. Be especially alert for signs of smoke inhalation and pulmonary damage — singed nasal hairs, mucosal burns, changes in the patient's voice, coughing, wheezing, soot in the mouth or nose, or darkened sputum. If necessary, assist with endotracheal intubation and administer 100% oxygen. When the patient's ABCs are stable, take a brief history of the burn and draw blood samples, as ordered, for diagnostic tests.

Next, stop residual burning and control bleeding. Remove any smoldering clothing. If material is stuck to the patient's skin, soak it with saline solution before you attempt to remove it. Remove all jewelry and any other constricting apparel. Then cover the burns with a clean, dry, sterile bed sheet. Remember, never cover large burns with saline-soaked dressings because this can drastically lower body temperature.

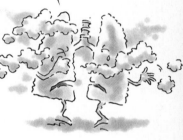

In the case of smoke inhalation, I may need you to administer 100% oxygen.

Solution resolution

Begin I.V. therapy, as ordered, to prevent hypovolemic shock and help maintain cardiac output. A patient with serious burns needs massive fluid replacement — especially during the first 24 hours after the injury. The practitioner may order a combination of crystalloids such as lactated Ringer's solution.

What goes in must come out

Closely monitor the patient's intake and output and check vital signs often. If the patient's limbs are badly burned, measuring blood pressure may be difficult; however, be sure to check blood pressure as required by applying a sterile nonstick pad to the area first. Finally, be prepared to assist in emergency escharotomy if the patient's burns threaten circulation.

Electrical burns

Tissue damage from electrical burns is difficult to assess because internal damage along the conduction pathway is commonly greater than the surface burn indicates. If possible, determine the voltage involved. This information helps the health care team assess possible internal damage more accurately.

Keep in mind that current passing through the body can induce ventricular fibrillation, cardiac arrest, or respiratory arrest — all life-threatening conditions requiring immediate intervention. (See *Electric shock*, page 92.)

Electric shock

When electric current passes through the body, the damage it does depends on:
• intensity of the current (measured in amperes)
• resistance of the tissues it passes through
• kind of current (alternating current, direct current, or a combination of both)
• frequency and duration of the current's flow.
    Electric current can cause injury in three ways:
• true electrical injury caused by current that passes through the body
• arc or flash burns caused by current that doesn't pass through the body
• thermal surface burns caused by associated heat and flames.
    The patient's prognosis depends on:
• site of the injury
• extent of damage
• his general health prior to the injury
• speed and adequacy of treatment.

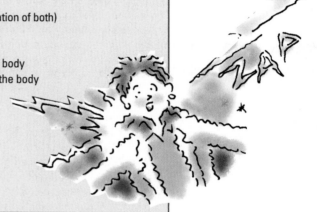

Chemical burns

When treating a patient with a chemical burn, begin by irrigating the wound with plenty of sterile water or normal saline solution for 30 minutes or more. Alkalis usually produce more severe burns than acids; however, the severity of the burn is usually determined by the length of time that the chemical was in contact with the patient's skin.

If the patient's eyes are involved, flush them with plenty of water or saline solution for at least 30 minutes. If it's an alkaline burn, irrigate until the pH of the cul-de-sacs returns to 7.0. Then have the patient close his eyes and cover them with dry, sterile dressings. Arrange for an ophthalmologic examination. Finally, note the type of chemical involved and the presence of any noxious fumes.

If the patient is to be transferred to a burn care unit soon after the accident, wrap him first in a sterile sheet and then a blanket for warmth and elevate the burned extremity to minimize edema.

Special considerations

Consider the following when caring for a patient with a burn:
• Assess the patient's level of pain, including nonverbal indications, and administer analgesics, such as morphine sulfate I.V, as ordered. (Avoid I.M. injections because tissue damage associated with the burn injury may impair drug absorption.)

• Keep the patient calm, provide periods of uninterrupted rest between procedures, and use nonpharmacologic pain relief measures, as appropriate.
• Administer histamine-2 receptor antagonists, as ordered, to reduce the risk of ulcer formation.
• Prepare the patient for possible grafting, as indicated.

Potential complications

Potential complications that may arise include:
• hypovolemic shock
• fluid overload
• pulmonary edema
• infection.
   Be sure to monitor the patient's vital signs and hemodynamic parameters and assess for signs and symptoms of infection, such as fever, elevated WBC count, and changes in burn wound appearance or drainage.

Skin grafting

Skin grafting may be necessary to repair defects caused by burns, trauma, or surgery. Depending on the graft's complexity, the procedure may be performed under local or general anesthesia and, in some cases, may be performed as an outpatient procedure. (For information on temporary skin grafts, see *Biological dressings*, page 94.)
   The surgeon may choose skin grafting as the preferred treatment option if:
• primary closure isn't possible or cosmetically acceptable
• primary closure would interfere with function
• the wound is on a weight-bearing surface of the body
• a skin tumor is excised and the site needs to be monitored for recurrence.
   Three types of skin grafts exist:
• split-thickness grafts — consisting of the epidermis and a small portion of the dermis
• full-thickness grafts — consisting of the epidermis and all of the dermis
• composite grafts — consisting of the epidermis, dermis, and underlying tissues (such as muscle, cartilage, and bone).

Secret of success

The success or failure of any skin graft depends on revascularization. Initially, a skin graft survives by direct contact with the underlying tissue, receiving oxygen and nutrients through existing

Dress for success

Biological dressings

Biological dressings function much like skin grafts, preventing infection and fluid loss and easing patient discomfort. However, biological dressings are only temporary measures because the body eventually rejects them. If the underlying wound hasn't healed, the dressing must be replaced with a graft of the patient's own skin.

Here's a comparison of the four types of biological dressings and their uses.

Type and source	Use and duration	Special considerations
Amnion Made from amnion and chorionic membranes	• Used to protect burns and to temporarily cover granulation tissue awaiting a graft • Must be changed every 48 hours	• Apply only to clean wounds. • Leave open to the air or cover with a dressing.
Biosynthetic Woven from man-made fibers	• Used to cover donor sites; to protect clean, superficial burns and excised wounds awaiting grafts; and to cover meshed grafts • Must be reapplied every 3 to 4 days	• Don't remove to treat the wound (biosynthetic dressings are permeable to antimicrobials).
Heterograft (xenograft) Harvested from animals (usually pigs)	• Used to protect granulation tissue after escharotomy, to protect excisions, to serve as a test graft before skin grafting, and to temporarily cover burns when the patient doesn't have sufficient skin for immediate grafting (Also used to cover meshed grafts, to protect exposed tendons, and to cover burns that are eschar-free and only slightly contaminated.) • Usually rejected in 7 to 10 days	• Dress or leave open. • Watch for signs of rejection.
Homograft (allograft) Harvested from cadavers	• Used for same purposes as a heterograft • Usually rejected in 7 to 10 days	• Observe the wound for exudate. • Watch for local and systemic signs of rejection.

blood vessels. However, the graft will die unless new blood vessels develop. For split-thickness grafts, revascularization usually takes 3 to 5 days; for full-thickness grafts, it may take up to 2 weeks.

Fall harvest

The graft is taken, or harvested, from an area of healthy tissue on the patient's body. Therefore, it's important to provide meticulous skin care to preserve potential donor sites. Also, because graft survival depends on close contact with underlying tissue, the recipient site — the wound — should be healthy granulation tissue that's free from eschar, debris, and infection.

Survival of the fittest

After a patient receives a skin graft, all aspects of care focus on promoting graft survival. Help the patient find comfortable positions for relaxing and sleeping that prevent him from lying on the area of the graft. If feasible, keep the graft elevated and immobilized. When needed, modify your routine to accommodate healing. For example, never use a blood pressure cuff over a graft site. In the case of a burn patient, omit hydrotherapy until the graft heals. Administer analgesics as necessary; however, remember to teach the patient techniques to reduce pain that don't involve medication (such as relaxation techniques).

Always use sterile technique when changing dressings and work gently to avoid dislodging the graft. Clean the graft site with a warm saline solution and cotton-tipped applicators, leaving the fine-mesh gauze over the graft intact. Aspirate any serous pockets. Change the gauze and apply the prescribed topical agent, as needed. Then cover the area with a gauze bandage.

There's no place like home

As the patient prepares to go home, discuss proper care with him. Explain that the dressings on the graft and donor sites shouldn't be disturbed for any reason. If he feels the dressing needs to be changed, he should call the practitioner and never attempt it himself. Emphasize that immobilizing the area of the graft is essential for speedy and complete healing. Later, as healing progresses, he can apply cream to the graft site several times a day to keep the skin pliable and help the scar mature.

Sun exposure can affect graft pigmentation. Explain this to the patient and suggest that he limit the amount of time he spends in the sun. Also suggest that he use sunblock anytime he plans to be outdoors.

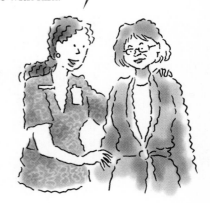

Be sure to teach your patient not to disturb the dressing on her graft and donor sites after she's discharged home.

Finally, almost all patients express concern about scarring and appearance. Explain that if scarring continues to be a problem when the graft completely heals, the patient can discuss plastic surgery options with his practitioner.

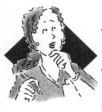

Quick quiz

1. After abdominal surgery, your patient says that he felt something "pop" when he was getting back into bed. You examine his wound and find bowel protruding. You should:

    A.   place the patient in high Fowler's position.
    B.   place the patient in low Fowler's position.
    C.   place the patient flat in bed.
    D.   place the patient on his left side.

Answer: B. Place the patient in low Fowler's position to reduce tension on the wound.

2. What's the first step in caring for a patient with a traumatic wound?

    A.   Get him to the hospital.
    B.   Take a blood pressure measurement.
    C.   Apply pressure bandages.
    D.   Assess his airway, breathing, and circulation.

Answer: D. Your first priority is to assess the patient's airway, breathing, and circulation.

3. When assessing your patient's burns, you note damage to the epidermis, dermis, and subcutaneous tissue. What type of burn has he suffered?

    A.   Superficial partial-thickness
    B.   Deep partial-thickness
    C.   Full-thickness
    D.   Deep full-thickness

Answer: C. In a full-thickness burn, the epidermis, dermis, and subcutaneous tissue are damaged. The burn may also involve muscle, bone, and interstitial tissue.

4. Your patient has deep partial- and full-thickness burn injuries to the posterior portion of both legs as well as his entire left and right arms. Using the Rule of Nines, what percentage of total BSA is involved?

    A.   18%
    B.   27%
    C.   36%
    D.   45%

Answer: C. The posterior portion of both legs constitutes 18% of BSA and the entire left and right arms constitute another 18%, for a total of 36%.

5. Which intervention can best protect the skin around a heavily draining surgical incision from irritation due to wound drainage?

    A.   Pouching the wound.
    B.   Applying packing and gauze dressings.
    C.   Applying a hydrocolloid dressing.
    D.   Applying an occlusive dressing.

Answer: A. Pouching prevents irritation of surrounding tissue when there's copious drainage from an incision.

6. To prevent skin tears, you should:

    A.   encourage the patient to wear short-sleeve tops.
    B.   use adhesive tape on dressings.
    C.   tell the patient to avoid sudden movements.
    D.   avoid using skin lotion.

Answer: C. Encourage your patient to avoid sudden or brusque movements that can pull the skin and possibly cause a skin tear.

7. Your patient has a surgical wound that has been closed for 8 days. During your wound assessment, you palpate a ridge along the incision line. This ridge may indicate:

    A.   normal healing.
    B.   wound dehiscence.
    C.   wound evisceration.
    D.   wound tunneling.

Answer: A. This ridge, known as the *healing ridge,* is a sign that normal healing is progressing.

Scoring

★★★ If you answered all seven questions correctly, strut your stuff! You've demonstrated an acute understanding of the chapter.

★★ If you answered five or six questions correctly, you deserve a hand! Your surgical approach to studying has served you well.

★ If you answered fewer than five questions correctly, that's okay! After a quick review, you'll be healed in no time.

5

Vascular ulcers

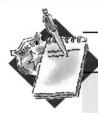

Just the facts

In this chapter, you'll learn:

♦ characteristics of venous, arterial, and lymphatic ulcers

♦ causes of vascular ulcers

♦ assessment criteria for vascular ulcers

♦ treatment options for vascular ulcers, including appropriate dressing types.

A look at vascular ulcers

The vascular system is composed of arteries, veins, capillaries, and lymphatics. Pressure from the beating heart carries blood away from the heart through the arteries into progressively smaller vessels until they connect with the capillaries. On the other side of the capillaries, small veins receive blood and pass it into progressively larger veins on its return trip to the heart. The lymphatic system is a separate system of vessels that collect waste products and deliver them to the venous system.

Disorders that affect the lymphatic vessels (blood vessels outside the heart) are known collectively as peripheral vascular disease (PVD). Vascular ulcers are chronic wounds that stem from PVD in the venous, arterial, and lymphatic systems. Venous and arterial ulcers are most common in the distal lower extremities, whereas lymphatic ulcers occur in the arms or the legs.

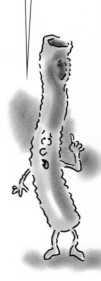

PVD has left a hole in my life.

Venous ulcers

Venous ulcers, which result from venous hypertension, occur on the lower leg. They affect about 1% of the population as a whole but are most common in older adults, affecting 3.5% of the population older than age 65. Venous ulcers account for 70% to 90% of all leg ulcers.

Venous anatomy and function

In the circulatory system, arteries carry blood away from the heart and veins carry blood back to the heart. Capillaries connect these two systems. On the venous side, venules are the small veins that receive blood from the capillaries and deliver it to the larger veins for its return trip to the heart.

Types of veins

In the lower portion of the body, where venous ulcers develop, there are three major types of veins: superficial veins, perforator veins, and deep veins.

Skin deep

Superficial veins lie just beneath the skin and drain into deep veins through perforator veins. Varicose veins are superficial veins that have become stretched and tortuous.

Central connectors

Perforator veins connect the superficial veins to the deep veins. Their name is derived from the fact that they perforate the deep fasciae as they connect superficial veins to the deep venous system.

U-turns

Deep veins receive venous blood from the perforator veins and return it to the heart. The major deep veins in the leg include the posterior tibial veins, anterior tibial veins, peroneal veins, and the popliteal veins. Each of these veins parallels a corresponding artery. (See *Major lower limb veins.*)

Vein walls and valves

Compared to arteries of the same size, veins have thinner walls and wider diameters. Vein walls have three distinct layers: an inner, endothelial layer (tunica intima); a middle layer of smooth muscle (tunica media); and an outer, supportive layer (tunica adventitia).

Veins also have a unique system of cup-shaped valves. The valves function to keep blood flowing in one direction—toward the heart. Deep veins have more of these valves than superficial veins, and veins in the lower leg have more of these valves than

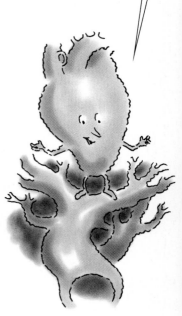

Miles of arteries, arterioles, capillaries, venules, and veins keep blood circulating from the heart to every functioning cell in the body — and back!

Major lower limb veins

Venous ulcers most commonly occur in the lower extremities. This illustration shows the major veins in this part of the body.

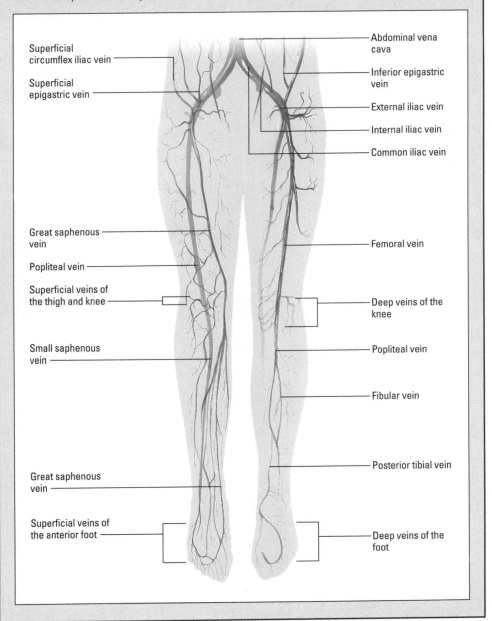

- Superficial circumflex iliac vein
- Superficial epigastric vein
- Great saphenous vein
- Popliteal vein
- Superficial veins of the thigh and knee
- Small saphenous vein
- Great saphenous vein
- Superficial veins of the anterior foot

- Abdominal vena cava
- Inferior epigastric vein
- External iliac vein
- Internal iliac vein
- Common iliac vein
- Femoral vein
- Deep veins of the knee
- Popliteal vein
- Fibular vein
- Posterior tibial vein
- Deep veins of the foot

A close look at a vein

This cross section of a vein clearly illustrates the three layers of the vein wall and its unique cup-shaped valves. These valves open toward the heart and, when closed, prevent blood from flowing backward.

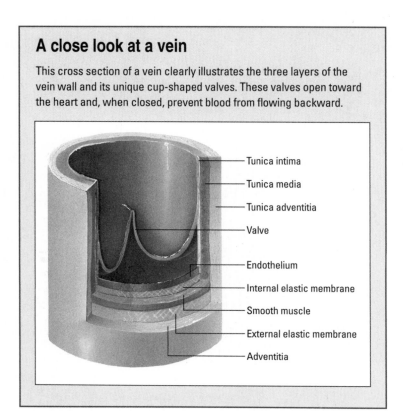

- Tunica intima
- Tunica media
- Tunica adventitia
- Valve
- Endothelium
- Internal elastic membrane
- Smooth muscle
- External elastic membrane
- Adventitia

veins in the thigh. In perforator veins, the valves open toward the deep veins. (See *A close look at a vein*.)

Pump it up!

Calf muscles have an important role in venous circulation. As calf muscles contract, they squeeze veins in the leg, forcing venous blood toward the heart. When they relax, veins in the leg expand and refill with blood from superficial and perforator veins. This pumping action is important because about 90% of venous blood travels to the heart this way. The other 10% of venous blood empties directly into the vena cava from the great saphenous vein. However, the calf muscles must be active for the calf muscle pump to work. Leg muscle paralysis or prolonged inactivity eliminates the calf muscle pump and inhibits venous blood flow.

Causes

Venous ulcers are the end stage of venous hypertension, which results from venous insufficiency (impaired flow of venous blood from the legs to the heart). In most cases, incompetent valves are to blame. Valve incompetency may be caused by a thrombus (blood clot) that renders the valve useless or by venous wall distention that separates valve cusps to the point where they no longer meet when the valve closes.

The pressure's rising

When the flow of venous blood slows, blood pools in the veins of the lower limbs and venous pressure rises. As the disease progresses, blood backs up through the perforator veins into superficial veins, causing varicose veins to develop in the superficial system. In many cases, edema develops as excess interstitial fluid accumulates. Keep in mind, however, that a patient with varicose veins may not have deep vein insufficiency; vascular tests can differentiate between these two problems.

Venous ulcers can occur in patients with superficial or perforator disease as well as those with deep vein disease. In all cases, the underlying problem is usually venous hypertension.

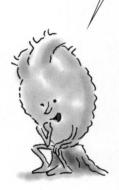

I think I get it! Venous insufficiency causes venous hypertension, which can cause venous ulcers.

Warning signs

Initially, venous ulcer development doesn't produce symptoms. The patient may report a general discomfort or aching in the affected areas.

Assessment

Proper assessment of venous ulcers includes collecting a thorough history and performing a physical examination.

History

Develop a complete history of the patient's experience with venous ulcers. Obtain answers to such questions as:
• When did the patient first notice the ulcer?
• Is this the first time that the patient has had an ulcer or is this a recurrence?
• If it's a recurrence, what type of treatment did the patient receive in the past? What type of pain management proved effective?
• Does the patient have a history of varicose veins? Venous thromboses? Arterial disease? Bleeding problems of any type? Leg trauma? Leg swelling?
• Does the patient use tobacco?

Physical examination

Record the size of the ulcer (length, width, and depth) and its location. Note any necrosis, drainage, or edema. Record the patient's description of pain associated with the ulcer. Pain may vary from nonexistent to extreme pain.

Venous ulcers may occur anywhere from the ankle to midcalf; however, they're most common on the medial aspect of the ankle above the malleolus and may extend all the way around the leg. Most have an irregular shape. The borders may have dry crusts or may be moist and slightly macerated from drainage. The ulcer itself is shallow with a base of beefy red granulation tissue. The surface may be covered by a yellow film or gray necrotic tissue. Black necrotic tissue is rarely present unless an acute injury has occurred. Check for edema and other signs of venous insufficiency. (See *Signs of venous insufficiency*.)

Taxed to the max

In venous insufficiency, red blood cells (RBCs), fluid, and fibrin leak into tissues. Note the color of the patient's skin. Hyperpigmentation is common even when ulcers aren't present. This color change is due to a buildup of hemosiderin in the interstitial tissue as the RBCs that have leaked into the tissue break down. The fibrin causes skin and subcutaneous tissue to thicken and become fibrotic — a condition called *lipodermatosclerosis*.

Signs of venous insufficiency

In a patient with venous insufficiency, check for ulcerations around the ankle. Pulses are present but may be difficult to find if edema is present. The foot may become cyanotic when dependent.

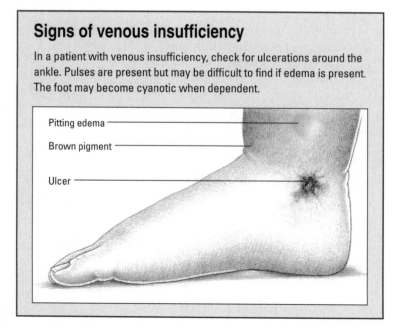

Pitting edema

Brown pigment

Ulcer

Keep a sharp eye

Other skin changes characteristic of venous insufficiency include edema, eczema, and atrophie blanche:

• Edema is one of the first signs of venous disease. It may be confined to the foot or the ankle or may involve the entire leg.

• Eczema is common, especially in patients who have recurrent ulcers. Skin over scar tissue and edematous tissue is fragile. Drainage from larger ulcers — or medications themselves — can irritate the skin and aggravate eczema.

• Atrophie blanche may appear as spots of ivory-white plaque in the skin, usually surrounded by hyperpigmentation. Some patients feel discomfort in these areas.

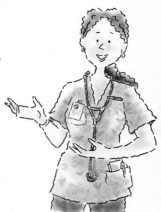

Watch for skin changes that are characteristic of venous insufficiency, including hyperpigmentation, edema, eczema, and atrophie blanche.

Diagnostic tests

Diagnostic tests for venous ulcers include plethysmography, venous duplex scanning, and venography.

Plethysmography

Plethysmography records changes in the volumes and sizes of extremities by measuring changes in blood volume. Types of plethysmography include:

• air plethysmography — which uses an inflatable pneumatic cuff placed around the limb to obtain volume measurements and standing and walking pressures

• photoplethysmography — which uses infrared light transmitted through the skin to measure venous reflux and filling times; delayed healing can be predicted by abnormal filling times

• strain-gauge plethysmography — which uses a mercury-filled, fine bore silicone rubber tube wrapped around the affected limb to measure blood flow and vascular resistance

• impedance plethysmography — which measures the change in resistive impedance of an electrical current as it passes through a body segment.

Venous duplex scanning

Venous duplex scanning is used to assess venous patency and reflux by measuring and recording venous pressures along an extremity as its veins are compressed and released. An experienced technician can use venous duplex scanning to identify thrombosis within a vein and determine whether it's acute or chronic as well as assess venous reflux and the status of valve function. The accuracy of the results may depend on the technician's skill.

Venography

Venography is the radiographic examination of a vein that has been injected with a contrast medium. In the past, this was the only test available to evaluate venous thrombosis; however, with the advent of newer noninvasive tests, venography is rarely used today.

Treatment

Effective treatment of a venous ulcer involves caring for the wound and managing the underlying venous disease. Controlling edema is the most important goal in managing chronic venous insufficiency. Methods to control edema include elevation of the affected limb, compression therapy and, sometimes, medication or surgery. Wound care involves selecting the best dressing for the venous ulcer.

Elevation of the limb

An effective method of reducing edema is to elevate the leg and allow gravity to drain fluid from it. This is best accomplished with the patient in bed with his legs elevated above the level of his heart. However, a patient with a cardiac or pulmonary condition may find this position intolerable. In this case, any elevation that the patient can tolerate is beneficial.

Compression therapy

Compression therapy is the most effective way of managing edema. Compression bandages are used when a patient can't elevate the affected limb. They're also helpful for times when a patient is on his feet. Various rigid and flexible types of compression bandages are available. However, before adding compression therapy to the patient's treatment regimen, assess his ankle-brachial index (ABI) to ensure the adequacy of arterial blood supply. (For more information, see "Ankle-brachial index," page 119.)

Unna's boot

A commercially prepared, inelastic, medicated gauze compression bandage, Unna's boot is one of the oldest treatments for venous ulcers. It's one of the most widely used compression bandages because it's inexpensive and effective. This dressing is especially useful for patients who pick at sores because it renders the ulcer inaccessible. The dressing should be changed weekly (or more frequently if needed).

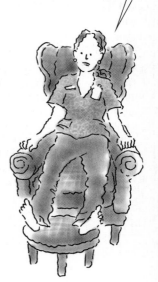

Get a leg up! The most effective method of reducing edema in a patient with venous ulcers is to raise the affected extremity higher than his heart.

Dress for success

How to wrap Unna's boot

To wrap an Unna's boot, follow these steps:
• Clean the patient's skin thoroughly and then flex his knee.
• With the patient's foot positioned at a right angle to his leg, wrap the medicated gauze bandage firmly— not tightly—around his foot. Make sure the dressing covers the heel.
• Continue wrapping upward, overlapping the layers by 50% with each turn. Make sure the dressing circles the patient's leg at an angle to avoid compromising his circulation. Smooth the boot with your free hand as you go, as shown in the top illustration.
• Stop wrapping about 1″ (2.5 cm) below the patient's knee, as shown in the bottom illustration. If constriction develops as the dressing hardens, make a 2″ (5.1-cm) slit in the boot just below the knee.
• If drainage is excessive, wrap a roller gauze dressing over the boot.
• Finally, wrap the boot with an elastic bandage in a figure-eight pattern.

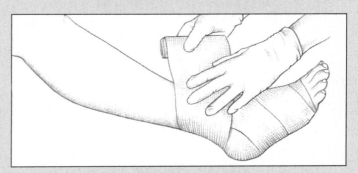

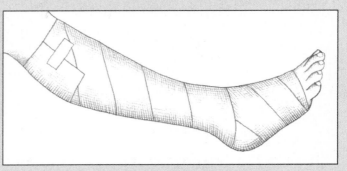

Unna's boot consists of a gauze roll that's impregnated with zinc oxide, calamine, and glycerin and placed over the skin from below the toes to just below the knee. Any concavity over the ulcer is filled with an additional dressing. This dressing is covered with cotton dressings to pad the wound and to absorb drainage. An elastic bandage is wrapped around the outside to provide compression. As the dressing dries, it becomes semirigid. (See *How to wrap Unna's boot.*)

In stiff pursuit

Although Unna's boot provides compression, protection, and a moist environment for healing, its most significant feature is its rigidity. Calf muscle contractions are key to the effectiveness of Unna's boot. As the patient walks, the rigid dressing restricts outward movement of the calf muscle, directing more of the contraction force inward and improving the function of the calf muscle pump and, in turn, venous circulation. Therefore, Unna's boot is much less effective for a sedentary or bedridden patient. If the patient finds the firmness against the ulcer uncomfortable, place a hydrocolloid or foam dressing over the ulcer before applying Unna's boot.

Compression stockings

Compression stockings are essential for long-term management of lower extremity venous disease. They're available in four classes of pressure, as measured at the ankle. Each package of stockings has a list of indications on the label; however, most health care professionals rely on their own experience when choosing a class for a patient based on his specific problem. Be aware that a patient with arthritis, back problems, or obesity may have problems putting on compression stockings.

CircAid Thera-Boot

If Unna's boot or compression stockings aren't viable options, a CircAid Thera-Boot may be the answer. This dressing provides about 30 to 40 mm Hg of compression and is easier to put on than compression stockings, as long as the patient can bend down to reach his legs. It can also continue compression even if there's a change in the size of the affected limb. The CircAid Thera-Boot is made of a nonelastic, semirigid material and has easy-to-use straps that secure the dressing in place. It's washable and reusable and can be removed at night and then put back on in the morning.

Layered compression bandages

Layered compression bandages with three or four layers are relatively new additions to the list of dressing options. In these bandages, the first layer is cotton wool, which protects the skin and absorbs moisture. This layer can be pulled apart and repositioned to fill concavities and create a more uniform fit. In some versions, a support bandage is the next layer. The support bandage provides a smooth surface for the compression layers above. Above this is a light compression bandage that provides about 17 mm Hg of pressure. The final layer is a compression bandage that provides 23 mm Hg of pressure.

Elastic bandages

Elastic bandages are inexpensive wraps that may be used for compression. They may be long-stretch or short-stretch.

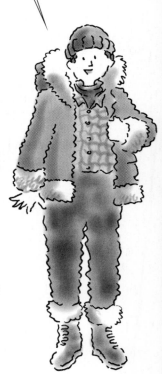

Sometimes layers are a must. Layered compression bandages protect the skin, absorb moisture, and provide compression.

The long...

A long-stretch bandage stretches to more than 140% of its length. Long-stretch bandages provide low working pressure and high resting pressure. A long-stretch bandage exerts a specific amount of pressure all the time, whether the patient is active or resting, and may provide more pressure than is desirable during periods of rest.

...and short of it

A short-stretch bandage has limited elastic stretch, typically less than 90% of its length. When stretched to its limit, a short-stretch bandage becomes semirigid, providing compression while the patient is active. When the patient rests, the dressing provides less compression, protecting his skin from unnecessary pressure. This type of bandage provides high working pressure and low resting pressure.

Graduated compression support stockings

As their name suggests, graduated compression support stockings provide a pressure gradient that's greatest at the ankle and lowest at the top of the stocking. This compression is consistent with the hydrostatic pressure in leg veins, which is greatest at the ankle and then diminishes up the leg. These stockings exert 100% of their pressure at the ankle, 70% at the calf, and 40% at the thigh level, producing a pressure gradient that helps reduce venous reflux. Knee-high length stockings are all that's necessary to treat edema caused by venous hypertension.

Compression pumps may be used in conjunction with support stockings. These devices are available with sleeves that intermittently inflate. They may have a single chamber or separate bladders that inflate sequentially.

Medication

Medications are rarely prescribed to treat venous ulcers. Antibiotics may be ordered to treat infection. In most instances, they're given systemically because topical antibiotics aren't effective in treating wound infections; in fact, they may interfere with healing. Also, if the patient is a candidate for skin grafting, topical antibiotics may be used to kill surface bacteria before the procedure.

Diuretics shouldn't be prescribed to treat edema in cases of venous insufficiency because edema is typically treated in these cases with compression and limb elevation. If the patient has concomitant heart failure, diuretics may be prescribed to treat it. Because diuretics can cause volume depletion and serious metabolic disorders, monitor the patient closely.

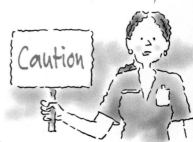

If diuretics are prescribed to treat a patient with concomitant heart failure, monitor the patient carefully for volume depletion and metabolic disorders.

Surgery

Venous ulcers are a chronic disorder that heal slowly and recur frequently. Consequently, surgery is rarely a viable treatment. Large surface defects may require repair by skin grafting; however, this is a temporary solution. The underlying problem of venous hypertension remains and, in time, edema beneath the scar tissue breaks down the scar and creates another ulcer.

Replacement parts

Valve transplant, which involves replacing a section of vein containing a defective valve with a section of vein containing a healthy valve, is performed selectively and almost never for a patient with venous ulcers. This is because, by the time an ulcer forms, venous disease is so pervasive that replacing a single valve won't help.

Success of SEPS

Another surgical procedure called *subfascial endoscopic perforator surgery* (SEPS) may be performed. SEPS is based on the theory that incompetent perforator veins cause ulcers at the ankles. During this procedure, faulty perforator veins are located and ligated, redirecting blood flow to healthy veins and improving ulcer healing.

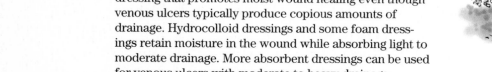

Be sure to choose the proper dressing for your patient with a venous ulcer. Now, if only choosing the right dress was that easy!

Wound care

Choosing the proper dressing is an important part of wound care because it affects wound healing. Occlusive dressings are typically selected for venous ulcers because they promote growth of granulation tissue and reepithelialization. If an ulcer contains necrotic debris, a moist gauze dressing or hydrocolloid dressing can be used to provide autolytic debridement. It's appropriate to select a dressing that promotes moist wound healing even though venous ulcers typically produce copious amounts of drainage. Hydrocolloid dressings and some foam dressings retain moisture in the wound while absorbing light to moderate drainage. More absorbent dressings can be used for venous ulcers with moderate to heavy drainage.

And introducing...

Newer therapies can also aid in healing chronic venous ulcers. Preliminary studies show that growth factors can be used to improve the healing rate in venous ulcers. In addition, two bioengineered skin equivalents (Apligraf and Dermagraft) can be used on venous ulcers that fail to heal within 4 weeks of treatment. (For more information on adjunctive therapies, see chapter 10, Therapeutic modalities.)

Arterial ulcers

Arterial ulcers, which are also called *ischemic ulcers,* are the result of tissue ischemia due to arterial insufficiency. They can occur at the distal (farthest) end of any arterial branch. Arterial ulcers account for 5% to 20% of all leg ulcers.

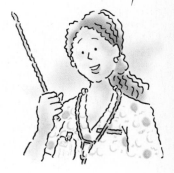

Arterial ulcers account for 5% to 20% of all leg ulcers.

Arterial anatomy and function

Like vein walls, artery walls have three layers:
• tunica intima (innermost layer) — composed of a single layer of endothelial cells on a layer of connective tissue
• tunica media (middle layer) — composed of a thick layer of smooth-muscle cells, collagen, and elastic fibers
• tunica adventitia (strong outer layer) — composed of connective tissue, collagen, and elastic fibers. (See *A close look at an artery.*)

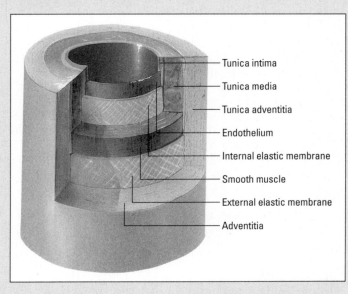

A close look at an artery

This cross section of an artery illustrates the layers that comprise the arterial wall.

- Tunica intima
- Tunica media
- Tunica adventitia
- Endothelium
- Internal elastic membrane
- Smooth muscle
- External elastic membrane
- Adventitia

With every beat of my heart

Arteries carry blood leaving the heart to every functioning cell in the body. Their strong, muscular walls allow expansion and relaxation with each heartbeat, smoothing the powerful pulse to an almost constant pressure by the time blood reaches the capillaries. The lower portion of the body receives its arterial flow through the abdominal aorta and the major arteries that branch from it. (See *Major lower limb arteries.*)

Causes

Arterial insufficiency occurs when arterial blood flow is interrupted by an obstruction or arterial stenosis (narrowing of an artery). Occlusion can occur in any artery — from the aorta to a capillary — and can result from trauma or chronic ailment.

The origins of occlusion

The most common cause of occlusion is atherosclerosis. Patients at highest risk for atherosclerosis include men, cigarette smokers, and individuals with diabetes mellitus, hyperlipidemia, or hypertension. Advanced age places patients at even greater risk. (See *Aging and arterial insufficiency.*)

Warning signs

In many cases, no signs of arterial insufficiency are apparent until the affected individual suffers an injury. As the demand for additional blood flow to the site of the injury outpaces an occluded artery's ability to deliver blood, ischemia occurs. Ischemia is a reduction in the flow of blood to any organ or body part. The primary symptom of ischemia is pain, which can be severe and may progress from claudication to rest pain.

Claudication

Claudication of the legs is similar to angina of the heart because the cause of both is an insufficient supply of oxygen. In the heart muscle, this oxygen deficiency causes the pain of angina. In leg muscles, the same deficiency causes the pain of claudication.

Claudication, which can occur in any muscle distal to a narrowed artery, is brought on by exercise and is relieved by rest. Typically, patients report claudication pain in the calf, thigh, or buttocks. It's measured by how many city blocks (or equivalent distance) the patient can walk before needing to stop to relieve the pain. Factors that tend to shorten the distance traveled before

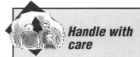

Handle with care

Aging and arterial insufficiency

When assessing elderly patients, be alert for signs of arterial insufficiency. As aging occurs, the tunica intima thickens and loses elasticity. Thickening of the intima is one cause of arterial stenosis, which puts older adults at greater risk for arterial insufficiency.

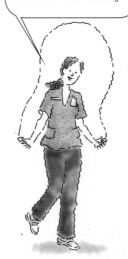

Claudication pain in the calf, thigh, or buttocks that's brought on by exercise and is relieved by rest may be the first sign of arterial insufficiency.

Major lower limb arteries

This illustration identifies the major arteries in the lower portion of the body.

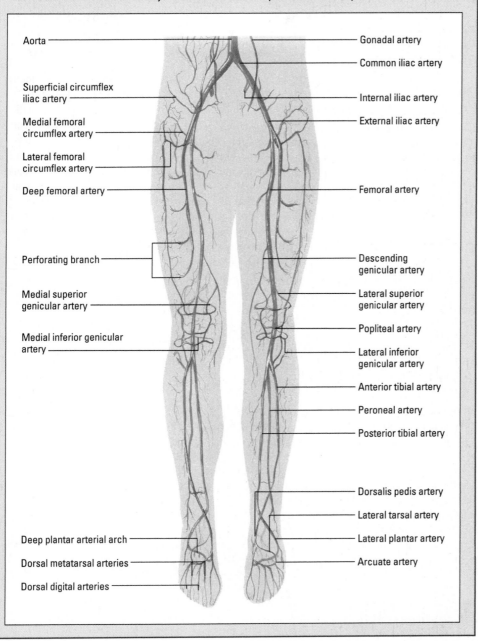

Aorta

Superficial circumflex iliac artery

Medial femoral circumflex artery

Lateral femoral circumflex artery

Deep femoral artery

Perforating branch

Medial superior genicular artery

Medial inferior genicular artery

Deep plantar arterial arch

Dorsal metatarsal arteries

Dorsal digital arteries

Gonadal artery

Common iliac artery

Internal iliac artery

External iliac artery

Femoral artery

Descending genicular artery

Lateral superior genicular artery

Popliteal artery

Lateral inferior genicular artery

Anterior tibial artery

Peroneal artery

Posterior tibial artery

Dorsalis pedis artery

Lateral tarsal artery

Lateral plantar artery

Arcuate artery

pain occurs include obesity, smoking, and progressive atherosclerotic disease.

Claudication occurs at a specific distance and is reproducible. Patients experiencing claudication don't have to sit or adopt a particular position to relieve the discomfort; merely stopping reduces the oxygen demand and relieves the pain. As arterial insufficiency progresses, the distance shortens until, ultimately, the patient feels pain even when resting.

Rest pain

Rest pain commonly occurs in the foot and can occur when the patient is asleep. Getting up and walking may provide some relief; however, walking isn't the key — lowering the extremity is. Gravity helps blood flow into the foot and calf, reducing the oxygen deficit and relieving discomfort. By the time rest pain occurs, tissues in the foot are severely ischemic, whether or not an ulcer is present. Unless arterial flow is restored, the patient may need amputation.

> Rest pain in the foot is more likely to be reduced by lowering the foot than by walking. Gravity helps blood flow into the foot, reducing the oxygen deficit and relieving discomfort.

Assessment

Assessment of arterial ulcers requires collecting a thorough patient history and performing a physical examination.

History

A patient history reveals whether the patient's wound is an arterial ulcer caused by arterial insufficiency. Obtain answers to such questions as:
• Has the patient experienced any pain?
• If he describes intermittent claudication, how far can he walk before pain sets in?
• If the patient says he has pain while resting, when did he first notice it and what measures does he take to relieve the pain?
• If the pain is in his foot, does getting up or hanging that foot over the edge of the bed help relieve the pain?
• What position is most comfortable for the patient? (Many patients spend their nights sleeping in a chair because the arterial pressure in the leg is too low to perfuse tissues while the leg is extended.)

Smoke signals

Ask the patient about smoking as well. If he smokes, determine how long he's been a smoker and how much he smokes.

Physical examination

Start your examination by inspecting the common sites of arterial ulcers: the tips of toes, the corners of nail beds on the toes, over bony prominences, and between toes. The edges of arterial ulcers are well demarcated. Because there's little blood flow to the tissue, the base of the ulcer is pale and dry with no granulation tissue present. You may see an area of wet necrosis or a dry scab. The skin surrounding the ulcer will feel cooler than normal on palpation. (See *Signs of arterial insufficiency.*)

Next, elevate the foot with the ulcer to a 30-degree angle; the skin color in an ischemic foot pales. Then ask the patient to place his foot in a dependent position. Ischemic skin becomes deep red as the tissue refills with blood. This dramatic color change is called *dependent rubor* — a sign of severe tissue ischemia. The nails may be thin and pale yellow, or they may have thickened due to an existing fungal infection in the nail beds. A Doppler signal may be heard over small arteries, but this doesn't signify blood flow that's sufficient enough to heal the ulcer.

Focus pocus

Perform a focused examination of the arterial system. Palpate the abdominal aorta for the presence of an aortic aneurysm. (In an obese patient, the abdominal aorta won't be palpable.) An embolus can occlude an artery and cause ischemia, and an aortic

---

Signs of arterial insufficiency

Arterial ulcers most commonly occur in the area around the toes. In a patient with arterial insufficiency, the foot usually turns deep red when dependent and the nails may be thick and ridged. In addition, pulses may be faint or absent; the skin is cool, pale, and shiny; and the patient may report pain in his legs and feet.

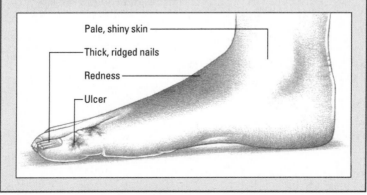

Pale, shiny skin

Thick, ridged nails

Redness

Ulcer

aneurysm may be the source of the embolus. "Blue toe syndrome" (a painful, ischemic toe) is caused by embolic debris in the arteries that supply the toe.

Palpate the femoral, popliteal, posterior tibial, and dorsalis pedis pulses in each leg and compare your findings. (See *Assessing lower extremity pulses.*) Keep in mind that an absent dorsalis pedis pulse may not be an abnormal finding. Under normal conditions, some patients don't have a palpable dorsalis pedis pulse. Pulses can be palpated when the pressure is about 70 mm Hg. If there's no palpable pulse, the pressure is probably less than 70 mm Hg. Pulses aren't palpable in a foot with an arterial ulcer.

Color chart

Compare the color of both legs to each other and palpate each leg for temperature. A difference in temperature of 10 degrees or more can be noted by palpation. While the patient lies down, elevate both of his feet about 12″ (30 cm) or to a 30-degree angle. Watch for a color change. Compress the great toe bilaterally and compare the capillary refill of each side. Normal tissue should refill in less than 3 seconds.

Diagnostic tests

Diagnostic tests commonly used to assess arterial flow to the extremities include segmental pressure recordings, Doppler ultrasonography, duplex ultrasonography, ABI, transcutaneous oxygen measurement, and arteriography.

Segmental pressure recordings

Blood pressure is the first test performed to assess the adequacy of arterial blood flow to the legs. Normally, blood pressure readings taken in the arm and the leg should be the same when the patient is lying down. A lower reading in the legs indicates an arterial blockage that may be caused by problems, such as a thrombus, cholesterol, or pressure on the outside of the artery.

Blood pressure is measured in both arms while the patient is lying down. Then blood pressure is measured at several points along each leg. Each reading is accompanied by a waveform tracing of the pulse. The entire procedure takes only 20 to 30 minutes. In some cases, the procedure is repeated after a short period of controlled exercise. In arterial insufficiency, arterial blood flow during exercise fails to keep up with muscle demand. Changes in the waveforms and Doppler signals should occur at the same time that the patient reports symptoms of claudication.

> Unequal blood pressure readings in your patient's arms and legs may alert you to problems with the blood flow to his legs.

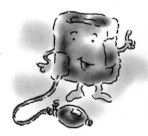

Assessing lower extremity pulses

These illustrations show where to position your fingers when palpating for pulses of the lower extremities. Use your index and middle fingers to apply pressure.

Femoral pulse

Press relatively hard at a point inferior to the inguinal ligament. For an obese patient, palpate in the crease of the groin, halfway between the pubic bone and the hip bone.

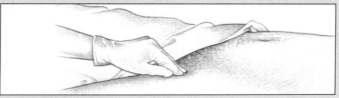

Popliteal pulse

Press firmly in the popliteal fossa at the back of the knee.

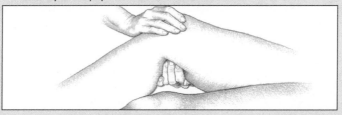

Posterior tibial pulse

Apply pressure behind and slightly below the medial malleolus.

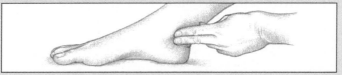

Dorsalis pedis pulse

Place your fingers on the medial dorsum of the foot while the patient points his toes down. The pulse is difficult to palpate here and may seem to be absent in healthy patients.

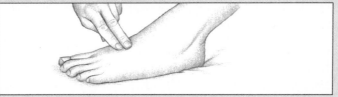

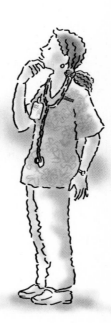

Doppler ultrasonography

In Doppler ultrasonography, sound waves are used to assess blood flow. This test may be used alone or in conjunction with other diagnostic tests to assess arterial blood flow. During the procedure, a handheld transducer directs high-frequency sound waves into the artery being tested. Sound waves that strike moving RBCs change frequency — a Doppler shift — in relation to the velocity of the RBCs. The practitioner then reviews the graphic record of these waveforms to determine whether an obstruction exists. (See *How the Doppler probe works.*)

How the Doppler probe works

The Doppler ultrasound probe directs high-frequency sound waves through layers of tissue. When the sound waves strike red blood cells (RBCs) moving in the bloodstream, the frequency of the sound waves changes in proportion to the velocity of the RBCs. A recording of these waves facilitates detection of arterial and venous obstruction.

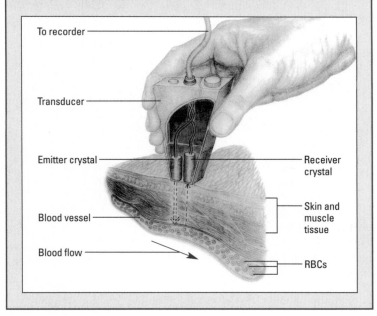

To recorder

Transducer

Emitter crystal

Receiver crystal

Skin and muscle tissue

Blood vessel

Blood flow

RBCs

(Text continues on page 119.)

Vascular ulcers

Vascular ulcers typically result from some form of peripheral vascular disease, which can affect the arterial, venous, and lymphatic systems.

Venous ulcers

Venous ulcers are the end stage of venous hypertension, which results from venous insufficiency. The most frequently occurring lower leg ulcers, venous ulcers are typically found around the ankle, as shown in the photo below.

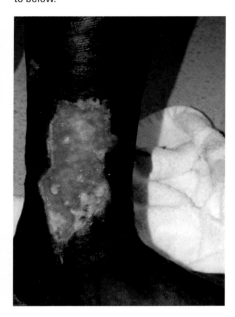

Lymphatic ulcers

Lymphatic ulcers result from lymphedema, in which thickened tissue compresses the capillaries. This occludes blood flow to the skin. These ulcers are extremely difficult to treat because of the reduced blood flow. The photo below shows a patient with lymphedema of the leg and a large lymphatic ulcer.

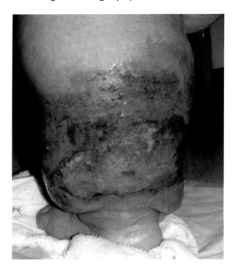

> Vascular ulcers differ in appearance and severity, depending on the part of the vascular system that's affected.

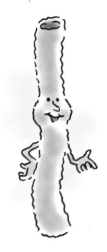

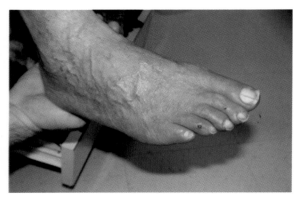

Arterial ulcers

Arterial ulcers result from insufficient blood flow to tissue due to arterial insufficiency. They're commonly found at the distal ends of arterial branches, especially at the tips of the toes, the corners of nail beds, or over bony prominences, as shown in the photo at left.

Staging pressure ulcers

You can use pressure ulcer characteristics gained from your assessment to stage a pressure ulcer, as described here. Staging reflects the anatomic depth of exposed tissue. Keep in mind that if the wound contains necrotic tissue, you won't be able to determine the stage until you can see the wound base. Currently, the National Pressure Ulcer Advisory Panel is evaluating the stage criteria.

Welcome hither, and learn thee of pressure ulcer stages. As Shakespeare knew, all the world's a stage...

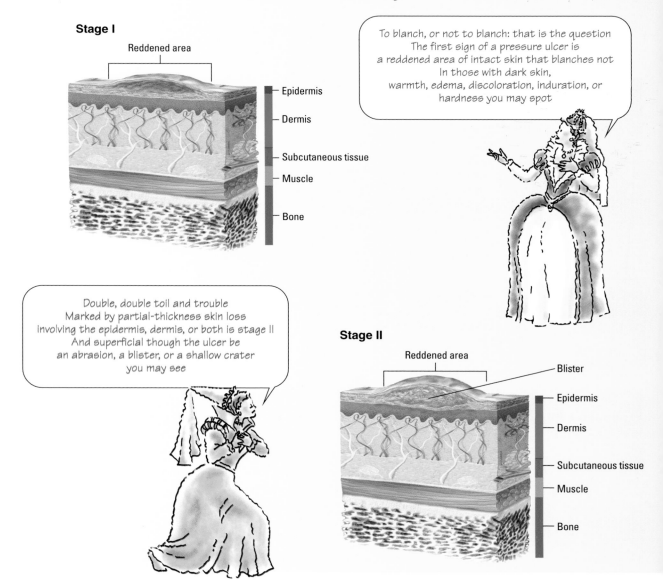

Stage I

Reddened area

- Epidermis
- Dermis
- Subcutaneous tissue
- Muscle
- Bone

To blanch, or not to blanch: that is the question
The first sign of a pressure ulcer is
a reddened area of intact skin that blanches not
In those with dark skin,
warmth, edema, discoloration, induration, or
hardness you may spot

Double, double toil and trouble
Marked by partial-thickness skin loss
involving the epidermis, dermis, or both is stage II
And superficial though the ulcer be
an abrasion, a blister, or a shallow crater
you may see

Stage II

Reddened area

- Blister
- Epidermis
- Dermis
- Subcutaneous tissue
- Muscle
- Bone

Stage III

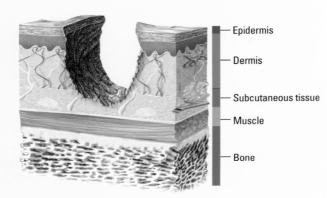

- Epidermis
- Dermis
- Subcutaneous tissue
- Muscle
- Bone

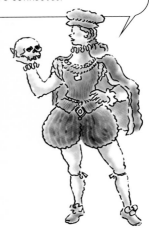

Now is the winter of our discontent
In stage III, the ulcer is a full-thickness wound
that appears like a deep crater when inspected
Underlying fasciae it may extend to
and thou might find undermining of the tissue
that's connected

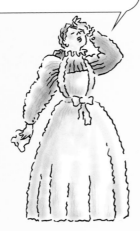

That it should come to this!
As through the skin the ulcer extends,
damage to muscle, bone, and supporting structures
accompany necrosis of tissues
Alas, undermining and sinus tracts
may also be issues

Stage IV

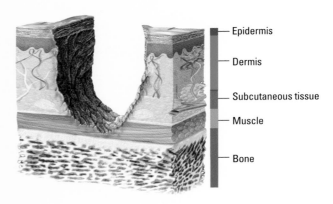

- Epidermis
- Dermis
- Subcutaneous tissue
- Muscle
- Bone

Parting is such sweet sorrow, that I shall say, "Go forth and provide
good wound care for all morrows!"

Diabetic foot ulcers

Because of the neurologic and vascular complications associated with diabetes, patients with this disorder are prone to foot ulcers. As with other pressure ulcers, diabetic foot ulcers typically develop over bony prominences when pressure is unrelieved.

This photo shows a patient with diabetes who has a pressure wound to the right lateral malleolus. Note the characteristic tissue changes associated with arterial insufficiency: thin, shiny skin; pale coloring; and muscular atrophy in the lower extremity.

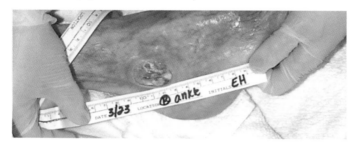

This photo shows a patient with type II diabetes who has developed a pressure ulcer from impaired protective sensation and poor mobility.

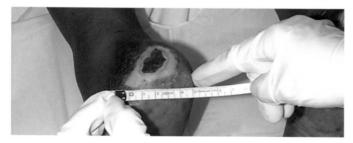

This photo shows a patient who has a diabetic foot ulcer on the plantar surface of the fifth metatarsal head. The circular shape of the wound is consistent with a wound created by pressure over a bony prominence.

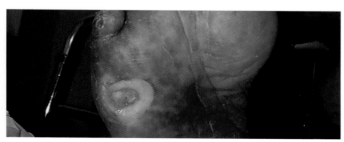

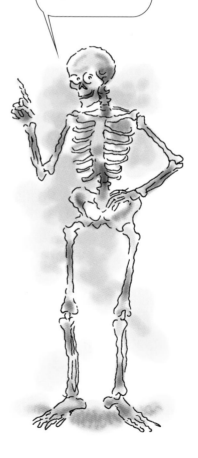

Pressure over bony prominences can cause all sorts of problems. For patients who have diabetes, the feet are at greatest risk.

Duplex ultrasonography

Similar to Doppler ultrasonography, duplex ultrasonography is used to measure blood flow in the arteries and veins of the legs and arms. A transducer probe with conductive gel is placed along different points of the vessel being studied and the data is viewed and recorded on an ultrasound monitor. Duplex ultrasonography can accurately identify areas of thrombosis in the blood vessels.

Ankle-brachial index

ABI is a value derived from blood pressure measurements that, taken as a whole, illustrate the progress of arterial disease — or degree of improvement — in the affected limb. Each value in the index is a ratio of a blood pressure measurement in the affected limb to the systolic blood pressure in the brachial arteries. Improvement, or lack thereof, becomes clear when the most recent value is compared to prior values.

The index can also be used to assess treatment methods. Comparing a reading taken before surgery, such as bypass surgery or angioplasty, to a reading taken afterward can indicate the procedure's effectiveness.

Take these steps

When measuring ABI, you'll use a Doppler ultrasound and a blood pressure cuff. The steps of the procedure are as follows:

Place the patient in a horizontal position so the brachial, dorsalis pedis, and posterior tibial arteries are at the same level.

Measure the brachial blood pressure on both sides. If they differ, use the higher of the two systolic pressures.

Wrap the blood pressure cuff around the patient's ankle, just above the malleoli. Identify the dorsalis pedis or posterior tibial artery and hold the Doppler transducer over the artery at a 45-degree angle.

Inflate the blood pressure cuff until you can no longer hear the Doppler signal; then slowly deflate the cuff. When the Doppler signal returns, record the pressure. This is the ankle systolic pressure.

Calculate the ABI by dividing the ankle pressure by the higher of the two brachial systolic pressures. (See *Interpreting ABI results*.)

Interpreting ABI results

This chart will help you interpret ankle-brachial index (ABI) calculations. Keep in mind that ABI results aren't reliable for patients with diabetes.

ABI	Interpretation
> 0.9	Normal
0.5 to 0.9	Claudication
0.2 to 0.5	Resting ischemic pain
< 0.2	Gangrene

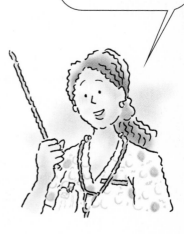

ABI is calculated by dividing ankle pressure by the higher of two brachial systolic pressures.

Transcutaneous oxygen measurement

Some vascular laboratories perform transcutaneous oxygen measurement to assess the perfusion of the microvasculature.

In this test, an electrode is attached to the patient's skin using double-sided tape. Room temperature is kept constant to ensure an accurate reading. Then the patient is monitored for about 20 minutes as the measurement is taken.

A transcutaneous oxygen of about 40 mm Hg is generally regarded as the cutoff value associated with inability to heal. However, the accuracy and, in turn, the dependability of this test varies depending on the laboratory and technician.

Arteriography

An invasive procedure that's only performed if the patient agrees to undergo a corrective procedure for any problem discovered, arteriography is performed by inserting a catheter into the arterial system, injecting a radiopaque contrast medium (a contrast medium that X-rays can't pass through), and taking an X-ray as the contrast medium is injected. The resulting image shows the lumen of the artery and any defect present.

The procedure has some disadvantages and significant risks. For example, several medications can't be taken for a time before the procedure. Also, some patients may be allergic to the contrast medium. Possible complications include injury to the artery, which requires emergency surgery, and hematoma, which requires drainage.

> The first treatment goal for arterial ulcers is to reestablish arterial flow. This can be achieved through bypass surgery or angioplasty and stents.

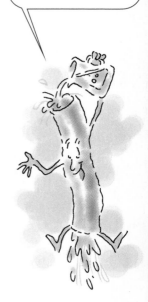

Treatment

The first goal in the treatment of an arterial ulcer is reestablishing arterial flow. Without oxygenated blood, the ulcer won't heal. Options for revascularization include arterial bypass surgery or angioplasty and stents. In addition, the ulcer must receive appropriate wound care. In general, medications aren't effective when arterial insufficiency has advanced to the point that ulcers are present.

Arterial bypass surgery

Arterial bypass is the gold standard for restoring arterial flow. The type and extent of bypass surgery depends on the ulcer's stage and location and the patient's general health. The graft may be autogenous (a vessel taken from the patient) or a synthetic material, typically Dacron or polytetrafluorene.

Angioplasty and stents

Less-invasive interventions, such as angioplasty, are more commonly used for treatment of arterial stenosis. During angioplasty, a catheter with a balloon is inserted into the patient's artery. Using fluoroscopy, the surgeon carefully maneuvers the catheter to the portion of the artery narrowed by plaque and then expands the balloon. The expanding balloon crushes the plaque against the wall of the artery, increasing the lumen diameter.

Stents are small metal structures that can be inserted into an artery after angioplasty to hold the artery open. They were developed to extend the amount of time that the artery remains open after angioplasty and reduce the need for surgery. Stent placement is gaining in popularity but the success rate of this procedure over time has yet to be determined. However, stents may be an alternative for a patient who's considered too high risk for surgery.

Wound care

Keep arterial ulcers dry and protected from pressure. For toe ulcers, place small alcohol pads between the toes and change them daily. As the alcohol dries, it promotes a dry ulcer bed. Never soak arterial ulcers. Ischemic tissue macerates in water, increasing the extent of tissue loss and promoting bacterial proliferation.

Foot fetish

Make sure the patient's foot is protected at all times. Consider using a large bulky dressing or protective footgear — there are many types to choose from. Keep in mind that ischemic tissue can easily develop additional ulcers with little irritation or pressure. Even pressure from the foot resting on the bed or an ill-fitting protective boot can initiate new ulcers. If your patient opts for foot protection, check the device carefully for possible pressure points.

If the ulcer area contains necrotic tissue or develops dry gangrene, continue to apply a dry dressing. Reassure the patient that a necrotic digit won't cause further harm. However, these areas have no sensation and must be protected from injury. If loss of a toe seems imminent, explain this to the patient and let him talk about his feelings. Having a necrotic toe fall off is a shocking and frightening event for most patients, but it's even more devastating when the patient isn't prepared for it.

Toe the line

Carefully monitor the line of demarcation between dead and viable tissues. This area is typically painful and easily infected. Treat infected ischemic tissue with I.V. antibiotics.

If revascularization succeeds, you'll need to change the type of dressing. At this point, you can treat the wound according to the

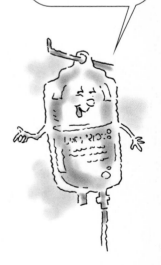

Ischemic tissue that becomes infected may need to be treated with I.V. antibiotics. That's why I'm hanging around!

axiom, "keep moist tissue moist and dry tissue dry," using any dressing that keeps the wound bed moist and the surrounding tissue dry. Consider using a hydrocolloid or hydrogel dressing. Use a moist dressing in the wound bed and cover this with a dry dressing for protection. When securing the dressing, remember to tape from one area of the dressing to another—not to the patient's skin.

Lymphatic ulcers

Lymphatic ulcers, which result from injury in the presence of lymphedema (swelling that results from impaired normal flow of lymph into venous circulation because of obstruction), occur most commonly on the arms and legs. Lymphedema leaves the skin vulnerable to infection and creates skin folds that trap moisture. These conditions cause ulcerations that become difficult to treat.

Lymphatic anatomy and function

The lymphatic system is a component of the peripheral vascular system. Lymph is a protein-rich fluid similar to plasma. As lymph circulates through lymphatic vessels, it collects wastes, including bacteria, and transports them to lymph nodes. The nodes filter wastes out of the lymph and add lymphocytes to the fluid. Lymph moves slowly through the lymphatic system, driven by muscle contraction and filtration.

Causes

Injury to the swollen tissue caused by lymphedema may result in an ulcer that's slow to heal.

Lymphedema may be congenital or acquired. Acquired lymphedema can be caused by surgery that severs or removes lymph nodes—radical mastectomy, for example—or it may result from compression of a vessel or node due to obesity or unrelated chronic swelling. For instance, patients with chronic venous hypertension and insufficiency may eventually develop lymphedema if venous edema is poorly managed.

Patients with lymphedema are prone to skin and soft tissue infections and may require long-term treatment with antibiotics. Prophylactic treatment with antibiotics is common because lymphedema causes progressive destruction of lymphatic vessels and nodes which, in turn, slowly increases the patient's risk of infec-

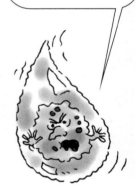

The lymphatic system circulates lymph through vessels to the lymph nodes, where wastes, including bacteria like me, are filtered out. And I didn't even say I was ready to leave!

tion. Recurrent cellulitis (tissue infection) is also commonly seen in patients with lymphedema.

Hard to handle

In the legs, lymphedema causes a steady seepage of fluids into interstitial tissue. In time, skin and underlying tissues become firm and fibrotic. Thickened tissue presses on the capillaries and occludes blood flow to the skin. The resulting poor circulation makes the leg ulcers that occur with lymphedema extremely difficult to treat.

Leg ulcers on lymphedematous tissue are usually the result of traumatic injury or pressure. However, in extreme cases of lymphedema, the folds of tissue develop deep fissures that trap moisture, causing tissue maceration and the start of a new ulcer. (See *Lymphatic ulcers and obesity*.)

Warning signs

The only warning sign of a lymphatic ulcer that a patient may report is a feeling of heaviness. This sensation is caused by edema in the affected extremity.

Assessment

Lymphatic ulcers are most common in the ankle area but may develop at any trauma site. Ulcers are shallow and may be oozing, moist, or blistered. The surrounding skin is usually firm, fibrotic, and thickened by edema. Cellulitis may be present as well. A diagnosis of lymphedema is based on the clinical appearance of the skin.

Handle with care

Lymphatic ulcers and obesity

Disorders, such as obesity, can induce venous hypertension. The patient who's morbidly obese may already have deep skin folds in which ulceration has developed. Pay close attention to these areas when assessing a bariatric patient for a lymphatic ulcer.

Diagnostic tests

Specific tests for determining whether a patient has a lymphatic ulcer don't exist; however, differentiating a lymphatic disorder from a vascular disorder can be difficult. Tests should be performed to rule out a vascular problem.

Treatment

Treatment of lymphatic ulcers has two goals: to reduce edema (and maintain the reduction) and to prevent complications such as infection. Leg elevation is an important part of therapy for patients with lymphedema. However, in cases of long-standing edema, elevation may be ineffective. The use of compression pumps and effective wound care are also part of the treatment plan.

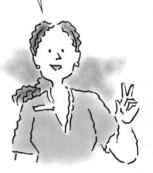

The two treatment goals for lymphatic ulcers are reducing edema and preventing complications such as infection.

Compression pumps

A compression pump is an effective method of reducing edema. Pump use is a lifelong part of managing edema. The pump reduces the volume of fluid in a lymphedematous limb. The pressure should be set low, in the range of 30 to 50 mm Hg. After each compression session, the patient must put on compression bandages or another compression garment. Without these, progress gained from the pumping is lost as soon as the patient stands or sits upright.

In addition, comprehensive decongestive therapy is a form of massage that has proven effective for some patients. After each session, the affected limb is wrapped with a short-stretch bandage. This therapy can be combined with compression pump use.

Wound care

Wound care for lymphatic leg ulcers is similar to care for venous ulcers. The primary difference is that the risk of infection is much higher for patients with lymphedema. In lymphedema, choose dressings that can manage large fluid loads while protecting surrounding skin, such as foams or other absorbent dressings.

Vascular ulcer care wrap-up

Keep the following tips in mind as you care for a patient with any form of vascular ulcer:

• The ulcer is only the tip of the iceberg. Care must also address the underlying disorder or the ulcer won't heal. For instance, with venous ulcers, the underlying venous hypertension must be treated. With arterial ulcers, arterial blood flow must be restored.
• Vascular disease is pervasive, so look for problems in other areas of the body.
• Be sure to choose the proper dressing for each ulcer. Remember, dressing choice depends on the characteristics of the ulcer as well as the ulcer type. (See *Dressings for vascular ulcers*, page 126.)
• For the most part, the wound care axiom of keeping moist tissue moist and dry tissue dry applies to vascular wounds. The one exception is an arterial ulcer, which must be kept dry until the area is revascularized. Then the axiom applies for arterial ulcers as well.
• Whenever possible, avoid using tape on the patient's skin. Skin affected by vascular disease is fragile and new ulcers form easily.

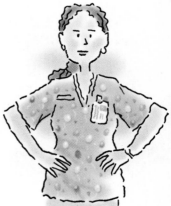

Remember to look for problems in other areas of your patient's body because vascular disease is pervasive.

Patient education

Typically, the success or failure of treatment is in the patient's hands because he has the primary responsibility for caring for this chronic condition. A motivated patient is more likely to adhere to the treatment regimen—a fact you should keep in mind as you prepare patient-teaching sessions. Patient teaching should provide clear instructions and rationales to encourage active patient participation.

Tips of the trade

Pass these tips along to the patient to promote vascular ulcer healing and reduce his risk of developing new ulcers:
• Look at your skin every day. Use lotion on dry, flaky skin.
• Use your calf muscles because frequent walks aid healing.
• Flex your feet up and down (as if you were using the gas pedal in a car) frequently when sitting.
• Elevate your legs whenever you sit.
• Wear shoes that fit well and always wear socks under shoes.
• Wear your compression stockings as directed.
• Don't sit or stand for long periods of time.
• Strive to maintain the agreed upon target weight.
• Report any skin injury to your practitioner.
• Don't smoke.

Dress for success

Dressings for vascular ulcers

Choosing the best type of dressing for your patient's vascular ulcer depends not only on the ulcer type but also on its condition. This chart lists indications and contraindications for each dressing according to ulcer type.

Dressing	Indications and contraindications		
	Venous ulcers	*Arterial ulcers*	*Lymphatic ulcers*
Alginate	• Use to manage copious drainage.	• Not indicated.	• Not indicated unless copious drainage is present.
Foam	• Use to protect the ulcer. • Use for absorption underneath a compression dressing.	• Use to protect the ulcer. • Use with dry gangrene. • Use for a moist, revascularized ulcer.	• Use to protect the ulcer. • Use to absorb drainage.
Gauze	• Use for absorption.	• Use for protection and to allow dry gangrene to maintain its dryness.	• Use for absorption or padding. (Don't allow it to dry out on the ulcer.)
Hydrocolloid	• Use to promote granulation. • Use to manage pain. • Don't use when copious drainage is present.	• Use for autolytic debridement. • Use for primary dressing after revascularization. • Don't use on ischemic tissue.	• Use to protect the skin. • Use to promote epithelialization. • Don't use when copious drainage is present. • Don't use when cellulitis is present.
Hydrogel	• Don't use when copious drainage is present.	• Use to maintain a moist wound bed. • Use to debride.	• Use to manage pain. • Use to debride.
Transparent film	• Not indicated.	• Use only after the ulcer is almost completely healed.	• Use to protect fragile skin. • Don't use when cellulitis is present.

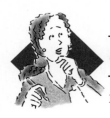

Quick quiz

1. Where's the most common site for a venous ulcer to develop?
A. Popliteal area
B. Anterior thigh
C. Lateral aspect of the foot
D. Medial aspect of the ankle

Answer: D. Venous ulcers are most common on the medial aspect of the ankle above the malleolus and may extend all the way around the leg.

2. Your patient has venous insufficiency. His leg edema is best treated by:
A. compression and leg elevation.
B. diuretics and compression.
C. leg elevation and diuretics.
D. restricting fluid intake and compression.

Answer: A. Compression helps to manage edema when the patient is upright. Leg elevation uses gravity to maximize venous return.

3. ABI is:
A. a guide to venous hypertension.
B. a value that reflects the amount of blood flow to the ankle.
C. obtained in a sitting position with feet flat.
D. normal if it's above 0.5 mm Hg.

Answer: B. In ABI, each value reflects the ratio of ankle systolic pressure to brachial systolic pressure.

4. The best dressing type for an ischemic ulcer on the toe is:
A. hydrocolloid.
B. wet to dry.
C. dry.
D. hydrogel.

Answer: C. An ischemic — or arterial — ulcer should be kept dry until blood flow to the area is restored.

5. Which sign or symptom is a key indication of progressive arterial insufficiency?

   A.   Cyanosis when the foot is in a dependent position
   B.   Pain
   C.   Edema
   D.   Hyperpigmentation of the skin

Answer: B. Pain is the most common presenting symptom in arterial disease with or without an ulcer.

6. Which therapy is the most effective treatment for managing edema?

   A.   Hydrotherapy
   B.   Compression therapy
   C.   Ice therapy
   D.   Diuretic therapy

Answer: B. Compression therapy is the most effective way to manage edema.

7. What test is performed first to assess arterial blood flow to the legs?

   A.   Segmental pressure readings
   B.   Doppler ultrasonography
   C.   Duplex ultrasonography
   D.   ABI

Answer: A. Segmental pressure readings is the first test performed to assess the adequacy of arterial blood flow to the legs.

Scoring

☆☆☆ If you answered all seven questions correctly, take a break! You deserve a splendid evening off tonight.

☆☆ If you answered five or six questions correctly, good for you! You're dancing right through these quizzes.

☆ If you answered fewer than five questions correctly, don't be upset! We're certain that your condition isn't chronic.

Pressure ulcers

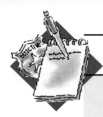

Just the facts

In this chapter, you'll learn:

♦ causes of pressure ulcers

♦ factors that increase pressure ulcer risk and ways to detect them

♦ ways to prevent pressure ulcers

♦ pressure ulcer assessment and staging criteria

♦ treatment options.

A look at pressure ulcers

Pressure ulcers are a serious health problem. Although incidence figures vary widely because of differences in methodology, setting, and subjects, data gathered through 10 years of nationwide studies reveal that 10% to 15% of the general population suffer from chronic pressure ulcers. Although this finding is significant in itself, prevalence in some groups—such as patients with spinal cord injuries, patients in intensive care units, and nursing home residents—is much higher.

At what cost?

Although prevalence statistics vary, what has become evident are the costs associated with pressure ulcers—the cost to patients in terms of suffering and diminished quality of life, the cost to the health care industry in terms of resources consumed and manpower hours to manage the problem, and the monetary cost to individuals, health insurers, and government agencies.

The problem is so acute that many insurers and government agencies now track outcomes to discern whether specific interventions help treat pressure ulcers and to encourage prevention, early intervention, and closer monitoring by the health care industry. Because a pressure ulcer is a chronic condition that's hard to

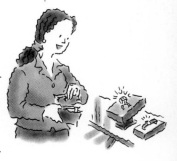

How much does this cost?! More important than money, pressure ulcers cost patients their quality of life.

heal and tends to recur frequently, prevention and early intervention are critical for more effective management.

Data OASIS

Data collected from Outcome and Assessment Information Set (OASIS) forms provide a basis for relating costs to clinical outcomes. The OASIS-B1 form is currently used by home health care agencies, as mandated by the Centers for Medicare and Medicaid Services.

The closer you get

Better disease management in pressure ulcer cases depends on closer collaboration among government agencies, insurers, and health care professionals. All involved are paying closer attention to prevention and the effectiveness of interventions, and they're finding better methods of quantifying and disseminating results. Soon, pressure ulcers will be a reportable condition for the Centers for Disease Control and Prevention. In addition, the health care objectives for the nation as a whole reflect a better understanding of the problem's severity. *Healthy People 2010* (a report of the nation's near-term health care goals) includes a goal of reducing by 50% the prevalence of pressure ulcers in nursing home residents.

Closed pressure ulcers

Although the pathology is the same, closed pressure ulcers are unique and potentially life-threatening pressure ulcers. They begin when shearing force causes ischemic necrosis in subcutaneous tissue. No surface defect marks this event and no signs of systemic infection are present. In time, pressure from inflammation in a necrotic debris cavity causes a small, unremarkable ulcer to form on the skin. This ulcer drains a large contaminated base.

Patients confined to wheelchairs because of spinal cord injury are at highest risk for this type of pressure ulcer, which occurs most commonly in the pelvic region. Prompt recognition is crucial.

A class of their own

Closed pressure ulcers can't be classified by stage or grade because it's impossible to determine the extent of damage until the defect is surgically opened. In addition, surgery that involves a wide excision and closure with a muscle rotation flap is the preferred and most expeditious treatment. However, other options should be explored before sacrificing muscle tissue because most flaps eventually fail.

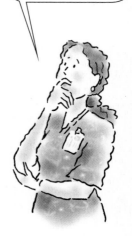

Closed pressure ulcers are unique and potentially life-threatening. Prompt recognition is difficult yet crucial.

Causes

Pressure ulcers are chronic wounds (wounds that fail to heal in a timely manner, resist treatment, and tend to recur) resulting from necrosis (tissue death) due to prolonged, irreversible ischemia brought on by compression of soft tissue. Technically speaking, pressure ulcers are the clinical manifestation of localized necrosis due to lack of blood flow in areas under pressure.

Shades of tolerance

Different tissues have different tolerances for compression. Muscle and fat have comparatively low tolerances for pressure, whereas skin has a somewhat higher tolerance. All cells, regardless of tissue type, depend on blood circulation for the oxygen and nutrients they need. Tissue compression interferes with circulation, reducing or completely cutting off blood flow. The result, known as *ischemia*, is that cells fail to receive adequate supplies of oxygen and nutrients. Unless the pressure relents, cells eventually die. By the time inflammation signals impending necrosis on the surface of the skin, it's likely that necrosis has occurred in deeper tissues.

Location, location, location

Pressure ulcers are most common in areas where pressure compresses soft tissue over a bony prominence in the body—the tissue is pinched between the outer pressure and the hard underlying surface. Other factors that contribute to the problem include shear, friction, and moisture. Planning effective interventions for prevention and treatment requires a sound understanding of pressure ulcer causes.

Pressure

Capillaries are connected to arteries and veins through intermediary vessels called *arterioles* and *venules*. In healthy individuals, capillary filling pressure is about 32 mm Hg where arterioles connect to capillaries and 12 mm Hg where capillaries connect to venules. Therefore, external pressure greater than capillary filling pressure can cause problems. In frail or ill people, capillary filling pressures may be much lower. External pressure that exceeds capillary perfusion pressure compresses blood vessels and causes ischemia in the tissues supplied by those vessels.

Tip of the iceberg

If the pressure continues long enough, capillaries collapse and thrombose and toxic metabolic by-products accumulate. Cells in

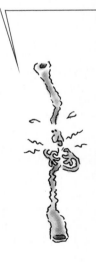

When external pressure exceeds capillary filling pressure, I become so compressed that ischemia may result.

nearby muscle and subcutaneous tissues begin to die. Muscle and fat are less tolerant of interruptions in blood flow than skin. Consequently, by the time signs of impending necrosis appear on the skin, underlying tissue has probably suffered substantial damage. Keep this in mind when assessing the size of a pressure ulcer.

The pressure mounts

When external pressure exceeds venous capillary refill pressure (about 12 mm Hg), capillaries begin to leak. The resulting edema increases the amount of pressure on blood vessels, further impeding circulation. When interstitial pressure surpasses arterial intravascular pressure, blood is forced into nearby tissues (nonblanchable erythema). Continued capillary occlusion, lack of oxygen and nutrients, and buildup of toxic waste leads to necrosis of muscle, subcutaneous tissue and, ultimately, the dermis and epidermis.

Spreading the load

The force associated with any given pressure increases as the amount of body surface exposed to the pressure decreases. For example, the force exerted on the buttocks of a person lying in bed is about 70 mm Hg. However, when the same person sits on a hard surface, the force exerted on the ischial tuberosities can be as much as 300 mm Hg. Consequently, bony prominences are particularly susceptible to pressure ulcers; however, they aren't the only areas at risk. Ulcers can develop on any soft tissue subjected to prolonged pressure. (See *Pressure points.*)

Pressure points

These illustrations show the areas at highest risk for ulcers when the patient is in different positions.

Sitting

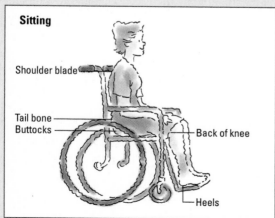

Shoulder blade

Tail bone
Buttocks

Back of knee

Heels

Lying

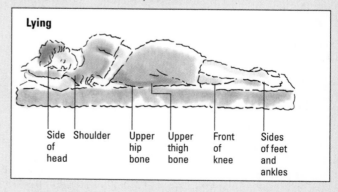

Side of head   Shoulder   Upper hip bone   Upper thigh bone   Front of knee   Sides of feet and ankles

Understanding the pressure gradient

In this illustration, the V-shaped pressure gradient results from the upward force exerted by the supporting surface and the downward force of the bony prominence. Pressure is greatest on tissues at the apex of the gradient and lessens to the right and left of this point.

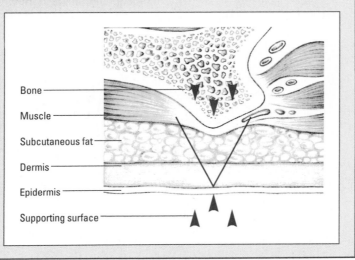

Bone

Muscle

Subcutaneous fat

Dermis

Epidermis

Supporting surface

Between a bone and a hard place

When blood vessels, muscle, subcutaneous fat, and skin are compressed between a bone and an external surface — a bed or chair, for instance — pressure is exerted on the tissues from both the external surface and the bone. In effect, the external surface produces pressure and the bone produces counterpressure. These opposing forces create a cone-shaped pressure gradient. (See *Understanding the pressure gradient.*) Although the pressure affects all tissues between these two points, tissues closest to the bony prominence suffer the greatest damage.

Under pressure

Over time, pressure causes a growing discomfort that prompts a person to change position before tissue ischemia occurs. In ulcer formation, an inverse relationship exists between time and pressure. Typically, low pressure for long periods is far more damaging than high pressure for short periods. For example, a pressure of 70 mm Hg sustained for 2 hours or longer almost always causes irreversible tissue damage, whereas a pressure of 240 mm Hg can be endured for a short time with little or no tissue damage. Furthermore, after the time-pressure threshold for damage passes, damage continues

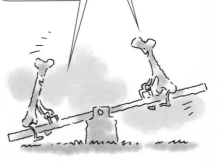

Did you know that we bones produce counterpressure when pressure is exerted on tissues from an external surface?

I don't know anything about that but I do know that if you don't exert some pressure right now, I'll be stuck up here all day!

even after the pressure stops. Although pressure ulcers can result from one period of sustained pressure, they're more likely to result from repeated ischemic events without adequate time between events for recovery.

Shear

Shearing force intensifies the pressure's destructive effects. Shear is a mechanical force that runs parallel, rather than perpendicular, to an area of skin; deep tissues feel the brunt of the force.

The shear truth

Shearing force is most likely to develop during repositioning or when a patient slides down after being placed in high Fowler's position. However, simply elevating the head of the bed increases shear and pressure in the sacral and coccygeal areas because gravity pulls the body down but the skin on the back resists the motion due to friction between the skin and the sheets. The result is that the skeleton (and attached tissues) actually slides somewhat beneath the skin (evidenced by the puckering of skin in the gluteal area), generating shearing force between outer layers of tissue and deeper layers. The force generated is enough to obstruct, tear, or stretch blood vessels. (See *Shearing force.*)

Shearing force reduces the length of time that tissue can endure a given pressure before ischemia or necrosis occurs. A sufficiently high level of shearing force can halve the amount of pressure needed to produce vascular occlusion. Research indicates that shearing force is responsible for the high incidence of triangular-shaped sacral ulcers and the large areas of tunneling or deep undermining beneath these ulcers.

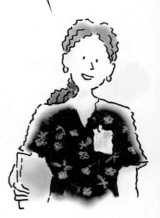

Be aware that a sufficiently high level of shearing force can halve the amount of pressure needed to produce vascular occlusion.

Friction

Friction is another potentially damaging mechanical force. Friction develops as one surface moves across another surface — for example, the patient's skin sliding across the bed sheet. Abrasions are wounds created by friction.

Friction prediction

Those at particularly high risk for tissue damage due to friction include patients who have uncontrollable movements or spastic conditions, patients who wear braces or appliances that rub against the skin, and older patients. Friction is also a problem for patients who have trouble lifting themselves during repositioning. Rubbing against the sheet can result in an abrasion, which increases the potential for deeper tissue damage. Elevating the head

Shearing force

Shear is a mechanical force parallel, rather than perpendicular, to an area of tissue. In this illustration, gravity pulls the body down the incline of the bed. The skeleton and attached tissues move, but the skin remains stationary, held in place by friction between the skin and the bed linen. The skeleton and attached tissues actually slide within the skin, causing skin to pucker in the gluteal area.

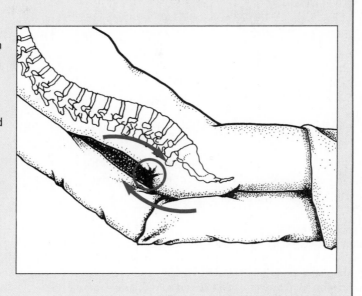

of the bed, as discussed earlier, generates friction between the patient's skin and the bed linen as gravity tugs the patient's body downward. As the skeleton moves inside the skin, friction and shearing force combine to increase the risk of tissue damage in the sacral area. Such dry lubricants as cornstarch and adherent dressings with slippery backings can help reduce the impact of friction.

Moisture

Prolonged exposure to moisture can waterlog, or macerate, skin. Maceration contributes to pressure ulcer formation by softening the connective tissue. Macerated epidermis erodes more easily, degenerates and, eventually, sloughs off. In addition, damp skin adheres to bed linen more readily, making the effects of friction more profound. Consequently, moist skin is five times more likely to develop ulcers than dry skin. Excessive moisture can result from perspiration, wound drainage, bathing, or fecal or urinary incontinence.

Are you calling me soft?

No. I'm really not. I'm just saying that prolonged exposure to moisture can soften connective tissue, which contributes to pressure ulcer formation.

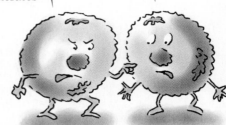

Risk factors

Factors that increase the risk of developing pressure ulcers include advancing age, immobility, incontinence, infection, poor nutrition, and low blood pressure. High-risk patients, whether in an institution or at home, should be assessed regularly for pressure ulcers.

Age

The risk of developing pressure ulcers increases with age because aging affects all aspects of healing. (See *Age and pressure ulcers.*)

Immobility

Immobility may be the greatest risk factor for pressure ulcer development. The patient's ability to move in response to pressure sensations as well as the frequency with which his position is changed should always be considered in risk assessment. Bariatric patients are especially at risk. (See *Pressure ulcers in bariatric patients.*)

Incontinence

Incontinence increases a patient's exposure to moisture and, over time, increases his risk of skin breakdown. Both urinary and fecal incontinence create problems as a result of excessive moisture and chemical irritation. Due to pathogens in the stool, fecal incontinence can cause more skin damage than urinary incontinence.

Handle with care

Age and pressure ulcers

With advancing age, the skin becomes more fragile as epidermal turnover slows, vascularization decreases, and skin layers adhere less securely to one another. Older adults have less lean body mass and less subcutaneous tissue cushioning bony areas. Consequently, they're more likely to suffer tissue damage due to friction, shear, and pressure. Other common problems that can contribute to pressure ulcer development in elderly patients include poor nutrition, poor hydration, and impaired respiratory or immune systems.

Infection

Although the role of infection in pressure ulceration isn't fully understood, animal studies on the effects of pressure and infection indicate that compression encourages a localized increase in bacteria concentration. Bacteria injected into animals localized at the compression site resulted in necrosis at lower pressures relative to the control group. Researchers concluded that compressed skin lowers local resistance to bacterial infection and that infection may reduce the pressure needed to cause tissue necrosis. Furthermore, researchers noted higher infection rates in pedicle flaps when denervation or loss of motor and sensory nerve function occurred. This may explain why neurologically impaired patients are more susceptible to infection and pressure ulceration.

Nutrition

Proper nutrition is vitally important to tissue integrity. A strong correlation exists between poor nutrition and pressure ulceration. Don't overlook the importance of nutrition during treatment.

Albumin acumen

Increased protein is required for the body to heal itself. Albumin is one of the key proteins in the body. A patient's serum albumin level is an important indicator of his protein levels. A subnormal serum albumin level is a late manifestation of protein deficiency. Normal serum albumin levels range from 3.5 to 5 g/dl. Serum albumin deficits are ranked as follows:
- mild—3 to 3.5 g/dl
- moderate—2.5 to 3 g/dl
- severe—less than 2.5 g/dl.

Pressure ulcer occurrence and severity are linked to malnutrition. One recent study found a direct correlation between pressure ulcer stage and degree of hypoalbuminemia (serum albumin level below 3.5 g/dl). Monitor the serum albumin levels of a high-risk patient and plan on nutritional intervention if he has hypoproteinemia.

Because of its short half-life (2 days), the prealbumin test is a more sensitive marker than albumin. It isn't as affected by liver disease and hydration status as albumin; however, it's more expensive to perform. A normal prealbumin value is 16 to 30 mg/dl.

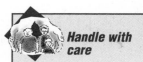

Handle with care

Pressure ulcers in bariatric patients

Bariatric patients are at risk for pressure ulcer development for several reasons:
- They're nutritional status may not be optimum.
- They're prone to developing protein malnutrition during metabolic stress (even though they may have excess body fat storage).
- They often have decreased vascularity in adipose tissue.
- They're unable to change position or move independently due to immobility.
- The moist environment in skin folds promotes bacterial growth, which can lead to fungal infections. (This decreased skin integrity also predisposes bariatric patients to pressure ulcer development.)

Blood pressure

Low arterial blood pressure is clearly linked to tissue ischemia, particularly in patients with vascular disease. When blood pressure is low, the body shunts blood away from the peripheral vascular system that serves the skin and toward vital organs to ensure their health. As perfusion drops, the skin is less tolerant of sustained external pressure and the risk of damage due to ischemia rises.

Risk factor assessment

Several assessment tools are available to help determine a patient's risk of pressure ulcers, including the Braden Pressure Sore Risk Assessment Scale — the most widely used pressure ulcer assessment tool — and the Norton scale. (See *Braden scale: Predicting pressure ulcer risk*, pages 140 and 141.) The Braden scale scores etiologic factors that contribute to prolonged pressure as well as factors that contribute to diminished tissue tolerance for pressure, including sensory perception, moisture, activity, mobility, nutrition, friction, and shear. The Norton scale assesses physical condition, mental state, activity level, mobility, and incontinence.

Common denominators

Most scales use the following factors to determine a patient's risk of developing pressure ulcers:
• immobility
• inactivity
• incontinence
• malnutrition
• impaired mental status or sensation.

Each category receives a value based on the patient's condition. The sum of these values determines the patient's score and level of risk. Scores for each category as well as the assessment as a whole help the health care team develop appropriate interventions. Most health care facilities require an assessment score for every patient admitted. The Agency for Health Care Research and Quality (AHRQ) *Guidelines for Pressure Ulcer Prediction and Prevention* recommends using either the Braden or Norton scale.

Early bird

In nursing home populations, most pressure ulcers develop during the 2 weeks immediately following admission, so early identification of at-risk patients is crucial. No definitive guidelines exist for how often to reassess a patient; however, use a common sense ap-

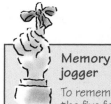

Memory jogger

To remember the five factors commonly used to determine a patient's risk of developing pressure ulcers, think of the five **I's**:

Immobility

Inactivity

Incontinence

Improper nutrition (malnutrition)

Impaired mental status or sensation.

proach, such as reassessing the patient when his condition changes or in the event that he becomes chair-bound or bedridden.

Prevention

Pressure ulcer prevention focuses on compensating for prevailing risk factors and addressing the underlying pathophysiology, including managing pressure, skin integrity, and nutrition. When planning interventions, be sure to adopt a holistic approach and consider all of the patient's needs.

Managing pressure

Managing the intensity and duration of pressure is a fundamental goal in prevention, especially for patients with mobility limitations. Frequent, careful repositioning helps the patient avoid the damaging repetitive pressure that can cause tissue ischemia and subsequent necrosis. When repositioning the patient, it's important to reduce the duration and intensity of pressure.

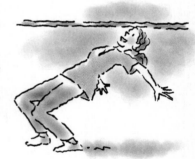

Your patient may not be quite ready to do the limbo yet but, remember, inactivity increases his risk of pressure ulcer development.

Positioning

Anytime you reposition the patient, look for telltale areas of reddened skin and make sure the new position doesn't place weight on these areas. Avoid the use of doughnut-shaped supports or ring cushions that encircle the ischemic area because these can reduce blood flow to an even wider expanse of tissue. If the affected area is on an extremity, use pillows to support the limb and reduce pressure. Avoid raising the head of the bed more than 30 degrees to prevent tissue damage due to friction and shearing force.

Baby steps

Inactivity increases a patient's risk of ulcer development. To the degree that the patient is physically able, encourage activity. Start with a short step—help him out of bed and into a chair. As his tolerance improves, help him walk around the room and then down the hall.

Positioning a patient in bed

When the patient is on his side, never allow weight to rest directly on the greater trochanter of the femur. Instead, have the patient rest his weight on his buttock and use a pillow or foam wedge to maintain the position. This position ensures that no pressure is placed

(Text continues on page 142.)

Braden scale: Predicting pressure ulcer risk

The Braden scale, shown here, is the most reliable of several existing instruments for assessing a patient's risk of developing pressure ulcers. The lower the score is, the greater the risk.

Patient's name ___*Harry Thompson*___ Evaluator's name ___*Beth Williams, RN*___

SENSORY PERCEPTION Ability to respond meaningfully to pressure-related discomfort	**1. Completely limited:** Unresponsive (doesn't moan, flinch, or grasp) to painful stimuli because of diminished level of consciousness or sedation OR Limited ability to feel pain over most of body surface	**2. Very limited:** Responds only to painful stimuli; can't communicate discomfort except by moaning or restlessness OR Has a sensory impairment that limits the ability to feel pain or discomfort over one-half of body
MOISTURE Degree to which skin is exposed to moisture	**1. Constantly moist:** Skin is kept moist almost constantly by perspiration, urine, etc.; dampness is detected every time patient is moved or turned	**2. Very moist:** Skin is often but not always moist; linen must be changed at least once per shift
ACTIVITY Degree of physical activity	**1. Bedfast:** Confined to bed	**2. Chairfast:** Ability to walk severely limited or nonexistent; can't bear own weight or must be assisted into chair or wheelchair
MOBILITY Ability to change and control body position	**1. Completely immobile:** Doesn't make even slight changes in body or extremity position without assistance	**2. Very limited:** Makes occasional slight changes in body or extremity position but can't make frequent or significant changes independently
NUTRITION Usual food intake pattern	**1. Very poor:** Never eats a complete meal; rarely eats more than one-third of any food offered; eats two servings or less of protein (meat or dairy products) per day; takes fluids poorly; doesn't take a liquid dietary supplement OR Is NPO or maintained on clear liquids or I.V. fluids for more than 5 days	**2. Probably inadequate:** Rarely eats a complete meal and generally eats only about one-half of any food offered; protein intake includes only three servings of meat or dairy products per day; occasionally takes a dietary supplement OR Receives less than optimum amount of liquid diet or tube feeding
FRICTION AND SHEAR	**1. Problem:** Requires moderate to maximum assistance in moving; complete lifting without sliding against sheets is impossible; frequently slides down in bed or chair, requiring frequent repositioning with maximum assistance; spasticity, contractures, or agitation leads to almost constant friction	**2. Potential problem:** Moves feebly or requires minimum assistance; during a move, skin probably slides to some extent against sheets, chair restraints, or other devices; maintains relatively good position in chair or bed most of the time but occasionally slides down

Date of assessment ___7/22/06___

3. Slightly limited: Responds to verbal commands but can't always communicate discomfort or need to be turned <div align="center">OR</div>Has some sensory impairment that limits ability to feel pain or discomfort in one or two extremities	**4. No impairment:** Responds to verbal commands; has no sensory deficit that would limit ability to feel or voice pain or discomfort	3
3. Occasionally moist: Skin is occasionally moist, requiring an extra linen change approximately once per day	**4. Rarely moist:** Skin is usually dry; linen only requires changing at routine intervals	3
3. Walks occasionally: Walks occasionally during day, but for very short distances, with or without assistance; spends most of each shift in bed or chair	**4. Walks frequently:** Walks outside the room at least twice per day and inside room at least once every 2 hours during waking hours	4
3. Slightly limited: Makes frequent though slight changes in body or extremity position independently	**4. No limitations:** Makes major and frequent changes in position without assistance	4
3. Adequate: Eats over one-half of most meals; eats four servings of protein (meat, dairy products) each day; occasionally refuses a meal, but usually takes a supplement if offered <div align="center">OR</div>Is on a tube feeding or TPN regimen that probably meets most nutritional needs	**4. Excellent:** Eats most of every meal and never refuses a meal; usually eats four or more servings of meat and dairy products; occasionally eats between meals; doesn't require supplementation	4
3. No apparent problem: Moves in bed and in chair independently and has sufficient muscle strength to lift up completely during move; maintains good position in bed or chair at all times		3
	TOTAL SCORE	21

Repositioning a reclining patient

When repositioning a reclining patient, use the Rule of 30, raising the head of the bed 30 degrees (as shown). Avoid raising the head of the bed more than 30 degrees to prevent buildup of shearing pressure. When you must raise it more — at meal times, for instance — keep the periods brief.

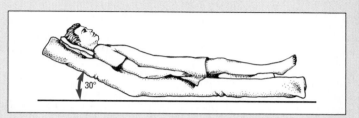

As you reposition the patient from his left side to his right side, make sure his weight rests on his buttock, not his hip bone. This reduces pressure on the trochanter and sacrum. The angle between the bed and an imaginary lateral line through his hips should be about 30 degrees. If needed, use pillows or a foam wedge to help the patient maintain the proper position (as shown). Cushion pressure points, such as the knees or shoulders, with pillows as well.

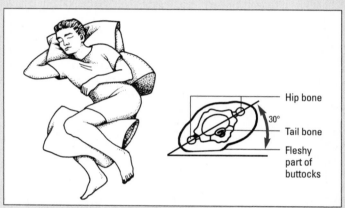

Hip bone

30°

Tail bone

Fleshy part of buttocks

on the trochanter or sacrum. Also, a pillow placed between the knees or ankles minimizes the pressure exerted when one limb lies atop the other. (See *Repositioning a reclining patient.*)

Suspending the heel is ideal

Heels present a particularly difficult challenge. Even with the aid of specially designed cushions, reducing the pressure on heels to below capillary refill pressure is almost impossible. Instead, suspend the patient's foot so that the bony prominence on the heel is under no pressure. A pillow or foam cushion placed under the patient's calves can permit a comfortable position while suspending his foot. Remember to take care to avoid knee contraction.

Positioning a seated patient

A patient is more likely to develop pressure ulcers from sitting than from reclining. Sitting tends to focus all of the patient's weight on the relatively small surface areas of the buttocks, thighs, and soles. Much of this weight is focused on the small area of tissue covering the ischial tuberosities. Proper posture and alignment help ensure that the weight of the patient's body is distributed as evenly as possible.

> Proper posture when sitting is a key part of pressure ulcer prevention.

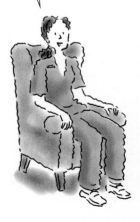

Proper posture preferred

Proper posture alone can significantly reduce the patient's risk of ulcers at the ankles, elbows, forearms, wrists, and knees. Be sure to include these points when explaining proper posture to the patient:

• Sit with your back erect and against the back of the chair, thighs parallel to the floor, knees comfortably parted, and arms horizontal and supported by the arms of the chair. (This posture distributes weight evenly over the available body surface area.)

• Keep your feet flat on the floor to protect your heels from focused pressure and distribute the weight of your legs over the largest available surface area—the soles.

• Avoid slouching, which causes shearing force and friction and places undue pressure on the sacrum and coccyx.

• Keep your thighs and arms parallel to ensure that weight is evenly distributed all along your thighs and forearms instead of being focused on the ischial tuberosities and elbows, respectively.

• Part your knees to keep knees and ankles from rubbing together.

Put your feet up

If the patient likes to use an ottoman or footstool, check to see if his knees are positioned above the level of his hips. If so, it means that his weight has shifted from the back of his thighs to the ischial tuberosities. The same problem—knees above hips—can occur if the chair itself is too short for the patient. In this case, recommend that he use a different footstool or chair.

Turn the other cheek

Patients at risk should reposition themselves every 15 minutes while sitting, if they can. Patients with spinal cord injuries can perform wheelchair pushups to intermittently relieve pressure on the buttocks and sacrum; however, this requires a fair amount of upper body strength. Others may have injuries that preclude using this technique.

Support aids and cushions

A pillow may be the first choice for a support aid but it's no longer the only option available. Today, you can also choose from a vast array of support surfaces and cushioning pads. Special beds, mattresses, and seating options that employ foams, gels, water, and air as cushioning agents make it possible to tailor a comprehensive and personal system of supports for the patient. Remember, effective care depends on knowledge of the classes and types of products available. (See *Pressure reduction devices*, page 144.)

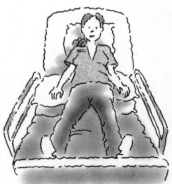

A pillow is always good for support but it isn't your only option.

Pressure reduction devices

Here are some special pads, mattresses, and beds that help relieve pressure when a patient is confined to one position for long periods.

Air-fluidized bed
Beads move under an airflow to support the patient, thus reducing shearing force and friction.

Alternating-pressure air mattress
Alternating deflation and inflation of mattress tubes changes areas of pressure.

Foam mattress or pads
Foam areas, which must be at least 3″ to 4″ (8 to 10 cm) thick, cushion skin, minimizing pressure.

Foot cradle
A foot cradle lifts the bed linens to relieve pressure over the feet.

Gel pads
Gel pads disperse pressure over a wide surface area.

Low-air-loss beds
Inflated air cushions adjust for optimal pressure relief for the patient's body size.

Mechanical lifting devices
Lift sheets and other mechanical lifting devices prevent shearing by lifting the patient rather than dragging him across the bed.

Padding
Pillows, towels, and soft blankets, when positioned properly, can reduce pressure in body hollows.

Water mattress or pads
A wave effect provides even distribution of the patient's body weight.

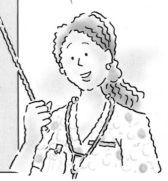

The more you learn about available options, the better prepared you are to best care for your patient.

False security

Be informed, but be cautious as well. Using these devices can instill a false sense of security. It's important to remember that as helpful as these devices may be, they aren't substitutes for attentive care. Patients require individual turning schedules regardless of the equipment used, and this schedule depends on your assessment of the patient's tolerance for pressure.

Horizontal support

Horizontal support surfaces include beds, mattresses, and mattress overlays. These products employ foams, gels, water, and air to minimize the pressure a patient experiences while lying in bed.

Beds

Specialty beds, such as oscillating and rotation beds, relieve pressure by rotating the patient or helping to lift the patient to reduce the risk of friction and shear. They also promote postural drainage and peristalsis. However, they're expensive and are rarely an option for a patient returning home.

Mattresses

Most mattresses worth considering use some form or manipulation of foam, gel, air, or water to cushion the patient. Foam core mattresses can provide the same benefits derived from a standard mattress with a foam overlay. Low-air-loss and high-air-loss mattresses are specialized support devices that pass air over the patient's skin. These mattresses promote evaporation and are especially useful when skin maceration is a problem. However, a risk of dehydration with the use of high-air-loss mattresses exists.

Water works

Water mattresses and some air mattresses use different media, but similar techniques, to evenly distribute pressure under the patient. Water mattresses use a gentle wave motion to maintain even distribution of pressure, whereas several types of air mattresses alternately inflate and deflate tubes within the mattress to distribute pressure.

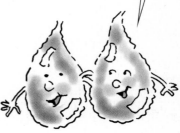

Water mattresses use a gentle wave motion to evenly distribute pressure.

Mattress overlays

The most common mattress overlays used in pressure ulcer prevention are foam, air, and gel overlays. Foam overlays should be at least 3″ (7.6 cm) thick for the average patient; thicker is even better. Although 2″ (5.1-cm) foam overlays may add comfort, they aren't suitable for patients at risk for pressure ulcers. Solid foam is preferable to the convoluted version. Be sure to select an overlay constructed from higher-quality foam because it will last longer.

Palm reading

If the patient's weight completely compresses a mattress overlay, the overlay isn't helping. To make sure the patient isn't bottoming out, hand check whenever a new overlay is put into service or if you suspect an overlay is breaking down. To hand check an overlay, slide one hand—palm up and fingers outstretched—between the mattress overlay and the mattress. If you can feel the patient's body through the overlay, replace the overlay with a thicker one or add more air to the mattress.

Vertical support

Products designed to help prevent pressure ulcers while sitting fall into two broad categories: products that relieve pressure and products that ease repositioning.

A cushy situation

Ambulatory and wheelchair-dependent patients should use seat cushions to distribute weight over the largest possible surface area.

Wheelchair-dependent patients require an especially rugged seat cushion that can stand up to the rigors of daily use. In many instances, a foam cushion that's 3″ to 4″ (7.5 to 10 cm) thick suffices.

Many wheelchair-seating clinics now use computers to create custom seating systems tailored to fit the physiology and needs of each patient. For patients with spinal cord injuries, the selection of wheelchair seating is based on pressure evaluation, lifestyle, postural stability, continence, and cost. Custom seats and cushions are more expensive; however, in this case, the added expense is justifiable. Encourage wheelchair-dependent patients to replace seat cushions as soon as their current one begins to deteriorate.

A position on repositioning

Repositioning is just as important when the patient is sitting as when he's reclining. For a patient requiring assistance, various devices are available, including overhead frames, trapezes, walkers, and canes. These devices can help the patient reposition himself as necessary. In addition, health care personnel can help maneuver I.V. poles and other support equipment.

Managing skin integrity

An effective skin integrity management plan includes regularly inspecting for tissue breakdown, routinely cleaning and moisturizing, and taking steps to protect the skin from incontinence, if applicable.

Inspecting the skin

Routinely inspect the patient's skin for pressure areas, depending on his assessed risk and his ability to tolerate pressure. Check for pallor and areas of redness—both signs of ischemia. Be aware that reactive hyperemia (redness that occurs after pressure is removed) is commonly the first external sign of ischemia due to pressure.

Cleaning the skin

Usually, cleaning with a gentle soap and warm water suffices for daily skin hygiene. Advise the patient to use a soft cloth to pat, rather than rub, his skin dry and to avoid scrubbing or using harsh cleaning agents.

Moisturizing the skin

Skin becomes dry, flaky, and less pliable when it loses moisture. Dry skin is more susceptible to ulceration. The number of skin moisturizing products available is truly staggering, so it shouldn't be hard to find one that the patient likes. The three categories of skin moisturizers are lotions, creams, and ointments. (See *Quick guide to moisturizers.*)

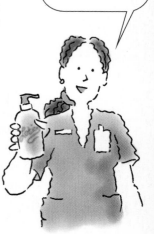

Three categories of skin moisturizers exist: lotions, creams, and ointments.

Quick guide to moisturizers

Keeping the skin moist is essential in helping to prevent pressure ulcer development, and many moisturizer products are available. Use this chart as a quick way to determine which product may be best for your patient.

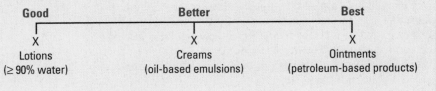

Good	Better	Best
X	X	X
Lotions	Creams	Ointments
(≥ 90% water)	(oil-based emulsions)	(petroleum-based products)

Lotions

Lotions are dissolved powder crystals held in suspension by surfactants. They have the highest water content, which is why lotions feel cool as they're applied. They also evaporate faster than any other type of moisturizer; consequently, they must be applied more often.

Creams

Creams are preparations of oil and water that are more occlusive than lotions. They don't have to be applied as often as lotions; therefore, three or four applications per day should be sufficient. Creams are better for preventing moisture loss due to evaporation than for replenishing skin moisture.

Ointments

Ointments are preparations of water in oil (typically lanolin or petroleum). They're the most occlusive and longest-lasting form of moisturizer. Studies indicate that petroleum is a more effective moisturizer than lanolin.

Protecting the skin

Although some moisture is good, too much can be a problem. Friction easily erodes waterlogged skin, making it more susceptible to irritants and bacteria colonization than dry skin. Close monitoring helps head off problems before they escalate.

Skin protection is particularly important if the patient is incontinent. Urine and feces introduce chemical irritants and bacteria as well as moisture, which can speed skin breakdown. To effectively manage incontinence, first determine the cause and then plan interventions that protect skin integrity while addressing the underlying problem.

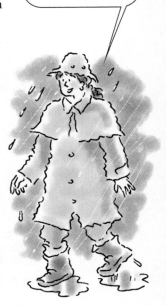

Be sure to protect your patient's skin from excessive moisture because waterlogged skin is more susceptible to bacteria.

In older adults, don't assume that incontinence is a normal part of aging. It isn't. Instead, consider factors that can precipitate incontinence, such as:
- fecal impaction and tube feeding (can cause diarrhea)
- a reaction to medication (can cause urinary incontinence)
- urinary tract infection
- mobility problems (can keep the patient from reaching the bathroom in time)
- confusion or embarrassment (can keep the patient from asking for a bedpan or help getting to the bathroom)
- clothing barriers, such as buttons or belts (can keep the patient from getting out of clothing in time).

Lend a helping hand

Whether the underlying cause is reversible, encourage the patient to ask for help when he needs a bedpan or needs to go to the bathroom. Use incontinence collectors, diapers or underpads, and skin barriers as appropriate to minimize skin damage. (See *Managing incontinence.*) Step up the frequency of mobilizing, toileting, inspections, cleansing, and moisturizing for these patients.

Managing nutrition

Proper nutrition, including a balanced dietary intake and maintaining proper weight, is essential to both ulcer prevention and healing.

Dietary intake

Protein is particularly important to skin maintenance. The patient needs a balanced diet that includes about 0.8 g/kg/day of protein. For most healthy adults, this means eating one or two 3-oz servings of protein each day in the form of meat, milk, cheese, or eggs.

Body weight

Low body weight is a problem for many pressure ulcer patients. An underlying illness or anorexia can make eating undesirable or impossible. To head off problems and to monitor the results of nutritional interventions, weigh the patient weekly; however, don't base your nutritional assessment solely on weight. Enemas or excessive water retention will increase or inflate the patient's weight. If the patient's history includes an unintentional weight loss of 10 lb (4.5 kg) or more during the previous 6 months, malnutrition may be the cause.

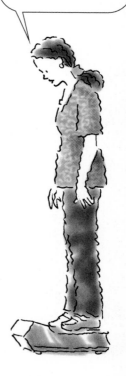

Be sure to weigh your patient weekly because low body weight is a problem for many pressure ulcer patients.

Managing incontinence

Patients experiencing incontinence require careful monitoring and special interventions to prevent skin damage caused by excessive moisture, chemical irritation, or microbial infection. Three types of aids can help you manage incontinence and minimize its impact on your patient: incontinence collectors, incontinence diapers and underpads, and topical barriers.

Incontinence collectors
• Condom catheters can help manage urinary incontinence in men (similar but less effective devices exist for women).
• Fecal incontinence collectors are pectin skin barriers with an attached, drainable pouch (similar to colostomy pouching systems).
• Collectors need to be changed on a regular schedule and whenever a leak is detected. Rectal tubes aren't a good alternative because they can cause complications, such as vasovagal response or ischemia of anal tissue.

Incontinence diapers and underpads
• Diapers and underpads wick moisture away from the patient's skin. Underpads and diaper alternatives include disposable absorbent gel diapers, disposable cellulose core diapers, and laundered reusable cloth diapers.
• Studies indicate that disposable gel diapers are significantly more effective in reducing wetness and maintaining normal skin pH than other alternatives. Reusable cloth diapers offer the least expensive alternative.

• Don't be tempted to put a plastic or paper linen saver under an incontinent patient; this holds moisture next to the patient's skin and compounds the problem.
• Don't secure the pad to the patient. Underpads work by absorbing wetness and allowing air to circulate over the skin, drying it.
• Diapers and underpads require routine monitoring so they can be changed promptly after urination or voiding.

Topical skin barriers
• Liquid copolymer film barriers protect intact skin from the damaging effects of incontinence. They're available in aerosol form or as disposable wipes. As they dry, these products form a strong, almost plasticlike barrier on the skin's surface that isn't easily washed off during normal cleaning.
• Paste is an excellent skin barrier. A paste is an ointment containing powder for thickness and durability that can be removed with mineral oil. Many pastes contain zinc oxide.

Assessment

Pressure ulcers can occur even with the best preventive measures. Effective treatment depends on a thorough assessment of the developing wound. Meaningful ulcer assessment requires a systematic and objective approach. First, gather the history of the ulcer, including etiology, duration, and prior treatment. Then your assessment should include information about the ulcer's:
• anatomic location
• characteristics (reactive hyperemia, blanchable and nonblanchable erythema)
• size (length, width, and depth in centimeters)
• base (necrotic, granulation, or epithelial tissue)

• drainage (amount and description)
• margins (sinus tracts, undermining, and tunneling)
• surrounding skin (redness, warmth, induration or hardness, swelling, signs of infection, wound edges).

Remember, in many cases, the full extent of ulceration can't be determined by visual inspection alone because there may be extensive undermining along fascial planes.

Pain drain

Before you examine the ulcer, assess the patient's pain. In most cases, pressure ulcers cause some degree of pain; in some cases, pain is severe. Have the patient rate his pain on a visual analog scale of 0 to 10, with 0 representing no pain and 10 representing severe pain. Similarly, ask the patient whether the pain interferes with his ability to function normally and, if so, to what degree.

Location

Ulcers are more common on the lower half of the body because it has more major bony prominences and more body weight than the upper half of the body. Two-thirds of pressure ulcers occur within the pelvic girdle.

Common locations for pressure ulcers include:
• sacrum
• coccyx
• ischial tuberosities
• greater trochanters
• elbows
• heels
• scapulae
• occipital bone
• sternum
• ribs
• iliac crests
• patellae
• lateral malleoli
• medial malleoli.

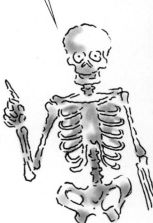

The areas over bony prominences are common pressure ulcer sites.

Characteristics

Tissue involvement ranges from blanchable erythema to the deep destruction of tissue associated with a full-thickness wound. Pressure against tissue interrupts blood flow and causes pallor due to tissue ischemia. If prolonged, ischemia causes irreversible and extensive tissue damage.

Reactive hyperemia

When the pressure that causes ischemia is released, skin flushes red as blood rushes back into the tissue. This reddening is called *reactive hyperemia*. A protective mechanism in the body dilates vessels in the affected area, which increases the blood flow and speeds oxygen to starved tissues. Reactive hyperemia first appears as a bright flush that lasts about one-half to three-quarters as long as the ischemic period. If the applied pressure is too high for too long, reactive hyperemia fails to meet the demand for blood and tissue damage occurs. Usually, reactive hyperemia is the first visible sign of ischemia.

Blanchable erythema

Erythema (redness) results from capillary dilation near the skin's surface. In the patient with pressure ulcers, this redness results from the release of ischemia-causing pressure. Blanchable erythema is redness that blanches (turns white) when pressed with a fingertip and then immediately turns red again when pressure is removed. Tissue exhibiting blanchable erythema usually resumes its normal color within 24 hours and suffers no long-term damage; however, it can signal imminent tissue damage. The longer it takes for tissue to recover from finger pressure, the higher the patient's risk of developing pressure ulcers.

In dark-skinned patients, erythema is hard to discern. Use bright light and look for taut, shiny patches of skin with a purplish tinge. Also, assess carefully for localized heat, induration, or edema, which can be better indicators of ischemia than erythema.

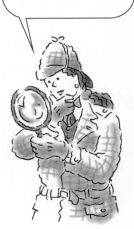

Erythema is often hard to discern in dark-skinned patients. Use a bright light to look for patches of skin that are taut, shiny, and purplish in color.

Nonblanchable erythema

In high-risk patients, nonblanchable tissue can develop in as little as 2 hours. The redness associated with nonblanchable erythema is more intense and doesn't change when compressed with a finger. Nonblanchable erythema can be the first sign of tissue destruction. If recognized and treated early, nonblanchable erythema is reversible.

Size

Using a disposable measuring tape, measure in centimeters the wound's length (longest dimension of the wound) and width (longest distance perpendicular to the length). Alternatively, carefully trace the wound margins on a piece of paper. In addition, a growing number of facilities now use wound photography.

Depth perception

Measure the ulcer's depth at its deepest point by inserting a gloved finger or a cotton-tipped swab. If you're using a probe other than your finger, be very careful; it's easy to cause further damage. Note any visible tunnels or undermining. If possible, use a gloved finger to gauge the extent.

The tissue in the ulcer base may be necrotic, granulation, or epithelial tissue.

Base

The type of tissue in the ulcer base determines the potential for healing and the type of treatment used. Know how to identify necrotic, granulation, and epithelial tissue.

Necrotic tissue

Necrotic tissue may appear as a moist yellow or gray area of tissue that's separating from viable tissue. When necrotic tissue is dry, it appears as thick, hard, and leathery black eschar. Areas of necrotic or devitalized tissue may mask underlying abscesses and collections of fluid. Before the ulcer can begin to heal, necrotic tissue, drainage, and metabolic wastes must be removed from the wound.

Granulation tissue

Granulation tissue appears as beefy red, bumpy, shiny tissue in the base of the ulcer. As it heals, a full-thickness ulcer develops more and more granulation tissue. Factors, such as tissue oxygenation, tissue hydration, and nutrition, can alter the color and quality of granulation tissue.

Epithelial tissue

Epithelialization is the regeneration of epidermis across the ulcer surface. It appears as pale or dark pink skin, first becoming evident at ulcer borders in full-thickness wounds and as islands around hair follicles in partial-thickness wounds. Wound healing can be assessed and quantified by the percentage of surface covered by new epithelium.

Drainage

Ulcers with drainage, or exudate, take longer to heal. Drainage characteristics include amount, color, consistency, and odor. Record the amount as scant, moderate, large, or copious. Describe the color and consistency together with clear, descriptive terms, such as:

- serous—clear, watery
- serosanguineous—clear red or reddish brown
- purulent—thick, yellow, cloudy.

The nose knows

Odor is a subjective observation—one that can suggest infection. It's important to clean the wound thoroughly before assessing the color and odor of drainage. Otherwise, perceived drainage may be a combination of dressing residue and dead cells—a combination that always produces a noxious odor. However, putrid odor that remains after wound cleaning may indicate anaerobic infection.

Margins

Pressure ulcer edges have distinct characteristics, including color, thickness, and the degree of attachment to the wound base.

Assess the epithelial rim as an integral part of the wound base. Ideally, there should be a free border of epithelial cells, which proliferate and migrate across the wound bed during healing. When epidermis at the ulcer edges thickens and rolls under, it impairs migration of epithelial cells. In epiboly, the wound edges thicken and the pressure ulcer becomes chronic, with little or no evidence of new tissue growth.

Tunnel troubles

In undermining, which occurs when necrosis of subcutaneous fat or muscle occurs, a pocket extends beneath the skin at the ulcer's edge. Tunneling differs from undermining in that both ends of a tunnel emerge through the skin's surface. In many cases, a tunnel connects two otherwise distinct pressure ulcers and it may be necessary to open the tunnel before the ulcer can heal.

Sometimes full-thickness pressure ulcers form tracts along fascial planes. When tracts are extensive, external palpation is the only way to determine their direction and length. If this is necessary, use a felt-tipped pen to outline the tract on the skin and measure the resulting image.

Surrounding skin

Assess intact skin surrounding the ulcer for redness, warmth, induration (hardness), swelling, and signs of infection. Palpate for heat, pain, and edema. The ulcer bed should be moist but the surrounding skin should be dry. The skin should be adequately moisturized but neither macerated nor eroded. Macerat-

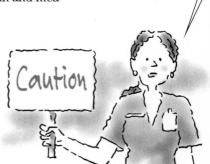

Watch for white, waterlogged skin around the wound's edges. This might indicate maceration.

Caution

ed skin appears waterlogged and may turn white at the wound's edges.

A saline-soaked dressing can cause maceration of surrounding skin unless the skin is protected. Other common causes of maceration include wound drainage and urine or feces contamination. Irritation or stripping may result from poor technique during dressing changes.

Staging

The most widely used system for staging pressure ulcers is the classification system developed by the National Pressure Ulcer Advisory Panel (NPUAP). This system, which defines four stages, has been adopted by the AHRQ Pressure Ulcer Guideline panels and is published in both sets of AHRQ *Clinical Practice Guidelines for Pressure Ulcers.* The NPUAP is currently evaluating the present staging system.

Now appearing on stage

Staging reflects the depth and extent of tissue involvement. Restaging isn't needed unless deeper layers of tissue are exposed by treatments such as debridement. Keep in mind that although staging is useful for classifying pressure ulcers, it's only one part of a comprehensive assessment. Ulcer characteristics and the condition of the surrounding skin provide equally important clues to the ulcer's prognosis.

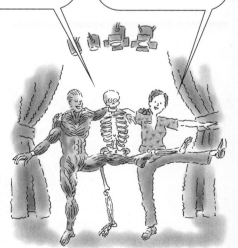

I thought this was a *real* musical. I think I need to have a talk with my manager...

Avoid stage four before your patient's out the door because he may be prone to lose skin, muscle, and bone!

Stage I

A stage I pressure ulcer is an area of skin with observable pressure-related changes when compared with an adjacent area of the same region on the other side of the body. Indicators include a change in one or more of these characteristics:
• skin temperature (warmth or coolness)
• tissue consistency (boggy or firm)
• sensation (pain or itching).

This ulcer presents clinically as a defined area of persistent redness in patients with light skin or persistent red, blue, or purple in patients with darker skin.

Stage II

A stage II pressure ulcer is a superficial partial-thickness wound that presents clinically as an abrasion, a blister, or a shallow crater involving the epidermis and dermis.

Stage III

A stage III pressure ulcer is a full-thickness wound with tissue damage or necrosis of subcutaneous tissue that can extend down to, but not through, underlying fasciae. The ulcer presents clinically as a deep crater with or without undermining of adjacent tissue.

Stage IV

A stage IV ulcer involves full-thickness skin loss with extensive damage, destruction, or necrosis to muscle, bone, and supporting structures (such as tendons and joint capsule). Undermining and sinus tracts may be present as well.

Complications

Complications, such as bleeding or infection, may develop during your care of a patient with a pressure ulcer. If an ulcer begins to bleed, apply pressure to the site. If the bleeding continues despite pressure, notify the practitioner. Be alert for foul-smelling drainage, a temperature over 101° F (38.3 °C), or erythema that increases on the skin surrounding the ulcer. If you notice any of these symptoms, notify the practitioner.

Treatment

Treatment of pressure ulcers follows the four basic steps common to all wound care:
• Debride necrotic tissue and clean the wound to remove debris.
• Provide a moist wound-healing environment through the use of proper dressings.
• Protect the wound from further injury.
• Provide nutrition essential to wound healing.
   A key element in all pressure ulcer treatment plans is identifying and treating, when possible, the underlying pathophysiology. If the cause of the ulcer remains, existing ulcers don't heal and new ulcers develop.

Typically, wound care involves cleaning the wound, debriding necrotic tissue, and applying a dressing that keeps the wound bed moist. Topical agents are used to resolve various issues. In addition, remember to teach the patient in order to improve the outcome of the treatment plan.

Wound cleaning

Wound cleaning removes wound debris, old dressing materials, and necrotic tissue from the wound surface. Pressurized wound irrigation is adequate for almost all wound cleaning. (For more information on wound cleaning, see chapter 3, Basic wound care procedures.)

Debridement

Debridement removes nonviable tissue and is the most important factor in wound management. Accurate staging and healing can't take place until necrotic tissue is removed. (For more information on debridement, see chapter 3, Basic wound care procedures.)

Dressings

Dressings serve to:
- protect the wound from contamination
- prevent trauma
- provide compression (if bleeding or swelling occurs)
- apply medications
- absorb drainage or debride necrotic tissue.

When choosing a dressing for a pressure ulcer, wound characteristics dictate the type of dressing you'll use. The dressing you select should protect wound integrity and keep the wound surface moist but prevent an excessive buildup of moisture, which can cause maceration and bacterial colonization. The frequency of dressing changes depends on the amount and type of wound drainage as well as the characteristics of the dressing.

Pack light

Wound cavities may require light packing or fill to prevent areas from walling off and developing into abscesses. Remember to be careful with packing because too much packing can generate more pressure and cause additional tissue damage.

Patient education

Remember that the goal of patient education is to improve the outcome. For any care plan to succeed after the patient leaves the hospital, he and his caregiver must understand the care plan, be physically and financially capable of carrying it out at home, and value both the information and the outcomes. Therefore, education and goal establishment should take into consideration the preferences and lifestyles of the patient and his family whenever possible.

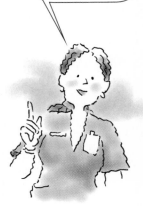

Remember, the goal of patient teaching is to improve the outcome.

Teach the patient and his family how to prevent pressure ulcers and what to do when they occur. (See *Pressure ulcer do's and don'ts.*) Explain repositioning and demonstrate what a 30-degree laterally inclined position looks like. If the patient needs assistance with repositioning, make sure he knows the types of devices available and where he can obtain them.

Mirror, mirror...

Show the patient how to inspect his back and other areas using a mirror. If he can't do this, a family member can help. Make sure he understands the importance of inspecting the skin over bony prominences for pressure-related damage every day.

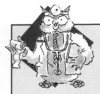

Get wise to wounds

Pressure ulcer do's and don'ts

With proper skin care and frequent position changes, patients and their caregivers can keep the patient's skin healthy—a crucial element in pressure ulcer prevention. Here are some important do's and don'ts to pass along to patients:

Do...
• Change position at least once every 2 hours while reclining. Follow a schedule. Lie on your right side, then your left side, then your back, then your stomach (if possible). Use pillows and pads for support. Make small turns between the 2-hour changes.
• Check your skin for signs of pressure ulcers twice daily. Use a mirror to check areas you can't inspect directly, such as the shoulders, tailbone, hips, elbows, heels, and back of the head. Report any breaks in the skin or changes in skin temperature to your practitioner.

• Follow the prescribed exercise program, including range-of-motion exercises every 8 hours or as recommended.
• Eat a well-balanced diet, drink lots of fluids, and strive to maintain the recommended weight.
• Use oil-free lotions.

Don't...
• Use commercial soaps or skin products that dry or irritate your skin.
• Sleep on wrinkled bed sheets or tuck your covers tightly into the foot of your bed.

If the patient needs to apply dressings at home, make sure he knows the proper ways to apply and remove them. Be sure to tell him where he can purchase supplies.

Nag about nutrition

Ensuring proper nutrition can be difficult but the patient and his family need to know how important proper nutrition is to the healing process. Provide materials on nutrition and maintaining an ideal weight, as appropriate. Show the patient how to create an easy-to-read chart of care reminders for home use.

In the name of progress

Pressure ulcers should be reassessed weekly. Measure progress by the reduction in necrotic tissue and drainage and the increase in granulation tissue and epithelial growth. Clean, vascularized pressure ulcers should show evidence of healing within 2 weeks. If they don't and the patient has followed the guidelines for nutrition, repositioning, use of support surfaces, and wound care, it's time to reevaluate the care plan.

The NPUAP has developed the Pressure Ulcer Scale of Healing (PUSH) tool that can be utilized to measure a wound's healing and response to interventions. Recent studies have shown that this tool is easy to use and reliable. It's a validated tool for assessing pressure ulcer healing rates. (For more information on the *PUSH tool*, see page 44.)

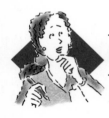

Quick quiz

1. Pressure ulcers are categorized as:
   A. acute wounds.
   B. chronic wounds.
   C. partial-thickness wounds.
   D. full-thickness wounds.

Answer: B. Pressure ulcers are chronic wounds.

2. A good way to assess your patient's pressure ulcer risk is to use:
   A. the PUSH tool.
   B. the Kransky Pressure Sore Assessment tool.
   C. your experience with other pressure ulcer patients.
   D. the Braden Pressure Sore Risk Assessment Scale.

Answer: D. The Braden Pressure Sore Risk Assessment Scale is used extensively to assess pressure ulcer risk.

3. Which intervention is most appropriate for preventing excessive heel pressure?
  A. Flexing the knees
  B. Placing a doughnut-shaped cushion under the feet
  C. Suspending the heels by placing a pillow under the calves
  D. Putting a pressure-reducing foam mattress under the heels

Answer: C. Suspending the heels using a pillow under the calves is the best way to protect heels from pressure ulceration.

4. Which body position simultaneously relieves pressure from the sacrum and trochanter?
  A. Prone
  B. Supine
  C. 30-degree lateral position
  D. 90-degree side-lying position

Answer: C. A 30-degree lateral position is the best way to relieve pressure from both the sacrum and the trochanter.

5. A pressure ulcer that appears innocent on the skin surface but conceals a deep, walled-off cavity filled with necrotic debris is a:
  A. closed pressure ulcer.
  B. stage II pressure ulcer.
  C. stage III pressure ulcer.
  D. stage IV pressure ulcer.

Answer: A. A closed pressure ulcer is a deep and potentially fatal lesion.

6. Which type of wound is created by friction?
  A. Contusion
  B. Laceration
  C. Ulcer
  D. Abrasion

Answer: D. Abrasions are wounds created by friction.

7. Which serum albumin level would be ranked as moderate?
    A.   2.2 g/dl
    B.   2.5 to 3 g/dl
    C.   3 to 3.5 g/dl
    D.   4 g/dl

Answer: B. A serum albumin level of 2.5 to 3 g/dl is ranked as moderate.

Scoring

☆☆☆ If you answered all seven questions correctly, congratulations! You've certainly demonstrated that you can handle the pressure.

☆☆ If you answered five or six questions correctly, nicely done! You're near the top of the pressure gradient.

☆ If you answered fewer than five questions correctly, don't despair! You'll reposition yourself soon.

Diabetic foot ulcers

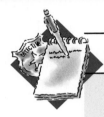

Just the facts

In this chapter, you'll learn:

♦ causes of diabetic foot ulcers

♦ prevention measures for diabetic foot ulcers

♦ assessment criteria for diabetic foot ulcers

♦ interventions for diabetic foot ulcer treatment.

A look at diabetic foot ulcers

Diabetes mellitus is a metabolic disorder characterized by hyperglycemia resulting from lack of insulin, lack of insulin effect, or both. Insulin transports glucose into cells, where it's used as fuel or stored as glycogen. Insulin also stimulates protein synthesis and storage of free fatty acids in fat deposits. An insulin deficiency compromises these important functions. Diabetes can begin suddenly or develop insidiously. (See *Diabetes: The not-so-sweet facts*, page 162.)

High plasma glucose levels caused by diabetes can damage blood vessels and nerves. Therefore, patients with diabetes are prone to developing foot ulcers due to nerve damage and poor circulation to the lower extremities. Good diabetes control may help prevent these potentially chronic problems or make them less serious.

Causes

Diabetic neuropathy, pressure and other mechanical forces, and peripheral vascular disease (PVD) can cause foot ulcers in patients with diabetes.

Diabetes: The not-so-sweet facts

Diabetes has been characterized as a modern day epidemic and it isn't hard to understand why when you look at the statistics for the United States:
• Diabetes is the seventh leading cause of death.
• Approximately 20.8 million people—7% of the population—have diabetes.
• Each year, practitioners diagnose 14.6 million new cases of diabetes.
• Diabetes occurs most frequently in African Americans, Hispanics, Asian Americans, and Native Americans, with middle-age and older adults at highest risk.
• Fifteen percent of all people with diabetes will develop diabetic foot ulcers.
• Between 14% and 20% of patients with diabetic ulcers require amputation.

Diabetic neuropathy

Peripheral neuropathy is the primary cause of diabetic foot ulcer development. Neuropathy is a nerve disorder that results in impaired or lost function in the tissues served by the affected nerve fibers. In diabetes, neuropathy may be caused by ischemia due to thickening in the tiny blood vessels that supply the nerve or by nerve demyelinization (destruction of the protective myelin sheath surrounding a nerve), which slows the conduction of impulses.

Polyneuropathy, or damage to multiple types of nerves, is the most common form of neuropathy in patients with diabetes. In the foot, a trineuropathy develops that includes:
• loss of sensation
• loss of motor function
• loss of autonomic functions (the autonomic nervous system controls smooth muscles, glands, and visceral organs). (See *Understanding diabetic trineuropathy*.)

Typically, impairment affects the feet and hands first and then progresses toward the knees and elbows, respectively. This presentation is called a *stocking and glove distribution*.

You've lost that warning feeling

As sensory nerves degenerate and die (sensory neuropathy), the patient experiences a burning or "pins-and-needles" sensation that might worsen at night.

As sensation declines, the patient risks foot injury. Impaired sensation prevents the patient from feeling stimuli, such as pain and pressure, that normally warn of impending damage. Anything from stepping on something sharp to wearing ill-fitting

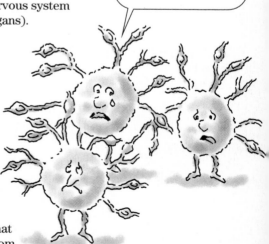

How tri-ing! The trineuropathy that commonly develops in the feet of diabetic patients includes loss of sensation, motor function, and autonomic function.

Understanding diabetic trineuropathy

Uncontrolled diabetes commonly results in a trineuropathy (three concurrent neuropathies) that dramatically increases a patient's risk of developing diabetic foot ulcers.

Sensory neuropathy

In sensory neuropathy, ischemia or demyelinization (see illustration below) causes nerve death or deterioration. When this occurs, the patient no longer feels painful stimuli and can't respond appropriately.

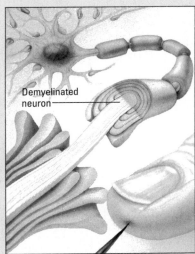

Demyelinated neuron

Motor neuropathy

In motor neuropathy, intrinsic muscles deep in the plantar surface of the foot atrophy, resulting in increased arch height and clawed toes. In addition, the fat pad that normally covers the metatarsal heads migrates toward the toes, exposing the metatarsal heads to more pressure and increasing pressure ulcer risk. The risk of ulcer development is high for the upper surfaces of clawed

toes as well, especially if the patient has poorly fitted shoes.

The illustration below shows the degenerative changes in the foot resulting from motor neuropathy. Shading indicates the areas where ulcers are most likely to develop.

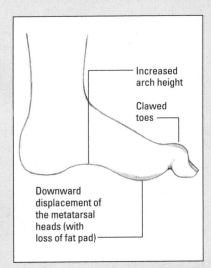

Increased arch height

Clawed toes

Downward displacement of the metatarsal heads (with loss of fat pad)

Autonomic neuropathy

In uncontrolled diabetes, autonomic neuropathy inhibits or destroys the sympathetic component of the autonomic nervous system, which controls vasoconstriction in peripheral blood vessels. The resulting unfettered flow of blood to the lower limbs and feet may cause osteopenia (reduction of bone volume) in foot and ankle bones.

In Charcot's disease (neuropathic osteoarthropathy), bones weakened by osteopenia suffer fractures that the patient doesn't feel due to sensory neuropathy. Over time, this process causes bony dissolution that culminates with the collapse of the midfoot into a rocker bottom deformity (see illustration below). Patients with Charcot's disease are placed on non-weight-bearing status until inflammation subsides.

Midfoot ulcers resulting from increased plantar pressures over the rocker bottom deformity heal slower than ulcers on the forefoot.

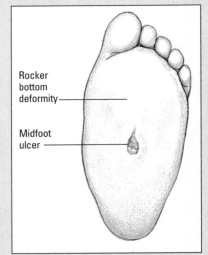

Rocker bottom deformity

Midfoot ulcer

shoes can result in foot injury because the patient can't feel the damage happening.

A-trophy that isn't a prize

As motor nerves degenerate and die (motor neuropathy), muscles in the limbs atrophy, especially the intrinsic muscles of the feet, which causes footdrop and structural deformities. These degenerative changes increase the patient's risk of stumbling or falling and further damaging the foot.

There's a bad infection on the rise

As autonomic nerves degenerate and die (autonomic neuropathy), sweat and sebaceous glands malfunction and skin on the patient's feet dries and cracks. If fissures develop, the risk of infection rises.

Mechanical forces

Mechanical forces that can cause diabetic foot ulcers include pressure, friction, and shear.

Pressure

Sensory neuropathy places a patient at increased risk for diabetic foot ulcers caused by pressure — especially a patient who's confined to a bed or wheelchair. Such a patient can suffer damage simply by letting his feet rest for too long on a bed or a wheelchair footrest. Impaired sensation prevents the patient from feeling the discomfort that results from staying in one position too long.

Prominent plantar pressure places

As with pressure ulcers, areas over bony prominences are the most common places for diabetic foot ulcers, including:
- metatarsal heads
- great toe
- the heel.

Friction and shear

Although pressure is the major mechanical force at work in the development of diabetic ulcers, it isn't the only one. Friction and shear can cause damage as well. A loose shoe rubbing against the foot or a foot sliding across a bed sheet can cause friction damage.

Shearly it's true

Shearing forces build up when damp skin sticks to a surface while the underlying bone and tissue move. For example, the skin of a

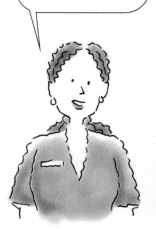

Remember that, along with pressure, friction and shear can also cause diabetic ulcers.

sweating foot can cling to a shoe while the underlying tissues slide beneath the skin.

Peripheral vascular disease

A common problem in patients with diabetes, PVD impairs the healing process of existing ulcers and may contribute to neuropathy as well. In PVD, atherosclerosis narrows the peripheral arteries, slowly reducing the flow of blood to the limbs. (See *How atherosclerosis impairs circulation.*) As perfusion drops, the risks of ischemia and tissue necrosis increase.

How atherosclerosis impairs circulation

In atherosclerosis, fatty deposits (cholesterol) and fibrous plaques accumulate along the walls of the arteries, narrowing the lumen and reducing the artery's elasticity. Thrombi (blood clots) form on the roughened surface of plaques and may grow large enough to block the artery's lumen.

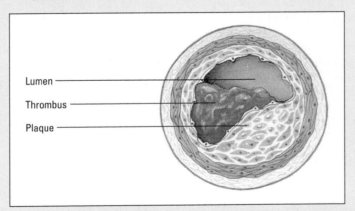

Lumen

Thrombus

Plaque

In diabetes, the arterial damage caused by atherosclerosis reduces blood flow to the lower limbs and to the nerves that innervate them. In addition to promoting ulcer development, poor perfusion slows the healing process for existing ulcers and impedes circulation of systemic antibiotics to infected areas.

Risk factors

Identifying the patient's risk factors is an important part of prevention. Loss of sensation is the single biggest risk factor but it isn't the only one. Here's a list of general risk factors for diabetic ulcers compiled by the American College of Foot and Ankle Surgeons:

- structural foot deformity (such as clawed toes, rocker bottom, or hallux vagus)
- trauma and improperly fitted shoes
- calluses
- prolonged, elevated pressure on areas of tissue
- limited joint mobility
- prolonged history of diabetes
- blindness or partial sight
- chronic renal disease.

Risk factors for diabetic foot ulcers may also be either local or systemic. Local risk factors include:

- previous foot ulcer or amputation
- neuropathy
- PVD.

Systemic risk factors include:

- age (older than age 65)
- hypertension
- hyperglycemia
- hyperlipidemia
- obesity.

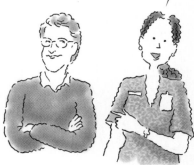

Teaching your patient how to eliminate or minimize diabetic ulcer risk factors is the best form of prevention.

Prevention

Diabetic ulcer prevention starts with identifying the patient's risk factors and then teaching him how to eliminate or minimize these risks.

Patient teaching

Teach the patient about ulcer care and prevention and the importance of controlling diabetes, including the consequences of not controlling it — for example, teach him that poorly controlled blood glucose levels can lead to peripheral neuropathy and vascular damage. Research indicates that tight glycemic control reduces the frequency and severity of neuropathy in patients with type 1 diabetes. Similar findings have been shown for patients with type 2 diabetes.

Teach the patient proper foot care and steps he can take to prevent ulcers, including daily examinations, skin washing and maintenance techniques, toenail care, and exercise. Also instruct him on how to choose proper socks and shoes. (See *Proper foot care.*)

A clean sock a day keeps the doctor away

White cotton-blended socks are the best choice for a patient with diabetes. Cotton-blended socks wick away moisture and allow air to circulate around the foot. White socks vividly show blood or exudate from an injury or ulcer that the patient may not feel. Regardless of the material, socks should always be nonconstricting and seamless over bony prominences. Socks with added padding can provide additional cushioning as well as some protection from shearing force.

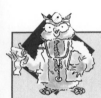

Get wise to wounds

Proper foot care

Here are some tips to teach your patient to help ensure proper foot care.

Performing foot hygiene
• Check your feet daily for injury or pressure areas (a long-handled mirror can help).
• Wash your feet with a mild soap and dry thoroughly between your toes.
• Check your bath water to make sure it isn't too hot (test the water with your elbow, if able; otherwise, use a thermometer or ask a family member to help).
• Apply a moisturizing cream to prevent dry, cracking skin on your feet and to balance skin pH. Don't apply moisturizer between the toes.
• Cut your toenails off squarely; see a podiatrist if they're dystrophic (deformed and thickened).
• Don't go barefooted—the risk of injury is too great.

Choosing socks
• Use silver ion-lined socks for fungus control.
• Wear white or light-colored socks in order to quickly detect bleeding from trauma.

• Wear natural fiber socks because they breathe better than synthetics.
• Wear socks that wick perspiration away from your feet (such as cotton-blended socks) to prevent maceration.
• Use diabetic padded socks for shear and friction control.

Choosing shoes
• Wear well-fitting shoes, not shoes that are too tight or loose.
• Wear shoes that breathe to reduce maceration and fungal infections.
• Wear new shoes for short periods (under 1 hour) each day initially; gradually increase the time as your feet adjust.
• If you have any foot deformities or a history of ulceration, wear professionally fitted shoes.
• Wash your shoes, if possible, to destroy microorganisms.
• Check your shoes before putting them on to make sure nothing fell in that could cause harm.

Team effort

Successful prevention programs for diabetic ulcers begin with health promotion. The patient should play an active role in setting personal health care goals, working in partnership with the health care team to achieve those goals.

Most patients with diabetes have multiple disorders, requiring a series of interventions involving many health disciplines — nurses, doctors, physical therapists, occupational therapists, nutritionists, podiatrists, endocrinologists, psychologists, diabetes educators, prosthetists or orthotists, and social workers.

Assessment

Assessment of diabetic foot ulcers includes gathering a thorough patient history and performing a physical examination and special testing of the lower extremities.

History

A thorough patient history is key to assessing diabetic foot ulcers. In addition to the basic information elicited during a traditional patient history, ask the patient about:
- date of onset of diabetes
- management measures
- glycemic control (using the glycosylated hemoglobin level as an indicator)
- medications
- other diagnosed problems (especially hypertriglyceridemia)
- status and history of any diagnosed neuropathy
- allergies, especially skin reactions
- tobacco and alcohol use
- recent changes in activity level
- date and location of previous ulcerations
- date that he first noticed the current ulcer
- the way in which the ulcer occurred
- type and quality of any associated pain.

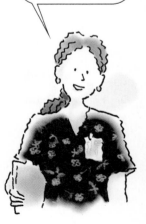

Treat the body as a unit, and remember, a thorough assessment of the patient's condition requires examination of several systems.

Physical examination

Use a holistic approach when performing the physical examination, which consists of a general examination and an examination of the patient's feet. Remember that the patient's overall physical health and state of mind affect wound healing.

General examination

During the general physical examination, you'll evaluate the patient's musculoskeletal, neurologic, vascular, and integumentary systems to provide perspective for assessing the condition of his lower limbs.

Bone up

Assess these aspects of the patient's musculoskeletal system:
• posture
• gait
• strength, flexibility, and endurance
• range of motion.

Make connections

Assess these aspects of the patient's neurologic system:
• balance
• reflexes
• sensory function.

Check the flow

Assess these aspects of the patient's vascular system:
• posterior tibial and dorsalis pedis pulses
• ankle-brachial index (ABI). (Keep in mind that ABI isn't as reliable due to calcification in the microvasculature.)

Get the skin-y

Assess these aspects of the patient's integumentary system:
• texture
• temperature
• color
• appendages (hair, sweat glands, sebaceous glands, nails).

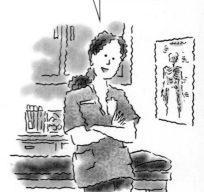

Be sure to check the high-risk areas of your patient's feet for evidence of ulcers.

Foot examination

Carefully examine the patient's feet to detect and assess foot ulcers. Check the following high-risk areas of the feet for existing or impending ulcers (calluses, for example):
• plantar surfaces (soles) of the toes
• tips of the toes
• area between the toes
• lateral aspect of the foot's plantar surface.

Wound characteristics depend on where the wound occurs on the foot. (See *Features of diabetic foot ulcers*, page 170.) Characteristics of surrounding skin may include:
• calluses (considered prewounds)
• blood blisters (hemorrhage beneath a callus)

Features of diabetic foot ulcers

In diabetic foot ulcers, characteristic clinical features depend on the ulcer's location.

Ulcer location	Clinical features
Plantar surface	Even wound margins
Great toe	Deep wound bed
Metatarsal head	Dry or low to moderate exudate
Heel	Low to moderate exudate
Tip or top of toe	Pale granulation with ischemia or bright-red, friable granulation tissue with infection

- erythema (a sign of inflammation or infection)
- induration (hardened edges)
- skin fissures (portals for bacterial entry)
- dry, scaly skin.

Special testing

Special tests provide a clearer picture of lower leg and foot health. These tests evaluate pressure, neurologic function, and perfusion. The results provide insight into the mechanism of injury, condition of the wound bed and surrounding tissue, prognosis for healing, and required treatment interventions.

Musculoskeletal tests

Harris mat prints and computerized pressure mapping are special musculoskeletal tests that provide information about the plantar pressures of the foot.

Harris mat prints

Pressure over bony prominences is one cause of diabetic foot ulcers. A simple method for determining areas of increased pressure on the plantar surface of the foot is to use an ink mat.

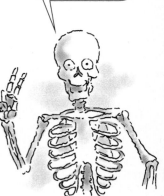

Harris mat prints and computerized pressure mapping are musculoskeletal tests that can aid you when assessing plantar pressures.

Making an impression

In Harris mat prints, the examiner inks the bottom of the mat, which has a grid to aid assessment of results, and places it on an evaluation template or clean sheet of paper. Then the patient steps on the uninked top surface of the mat, placing equal weight on each foot. If needed, the examiner holds the patient's outstretched hands to help ensure equal weight distribution. The impression on the template or sheet of paper shows relative areas of pressure under the patient's foot. Darker areas on the grid indicate high-pressure areas. In a case where a dynamic impression is required, the patient slowly walks across the mat to create the impression.

Under pressure

High-pressure areas usually correlate with calluses (prewounds) or existing wounds. The results help guide the choice of special off-loading devices, which help relieve pressure when the patient stands or walks.

Computerized pressure mapping

Computerized pressure mapping devices test plantar pressures while the patient is wearing a shoe and when he's barefoot. The approach is similar to Harris mat prints; however, in this test, a computer maps the pressures and displays the results on a print-out. A color gradient illustrates relative pressure, with red and orange indicating areas where pressure is highest.

Neurologic tests

Neurologic tests for the lower extremities include deep tendon reflexes testing, vibration perception testing with a tuning fork or biothesiometer, and Semmes-Weinstein monofilament testing for protective sensation.

Deep tendon reflexes testing

Peripheral neuropathy causes a decrease in deep tendon reflexes. Decreased deep tendon reflexes correlate with muscular atrophy, usually the intrinsic muscles of the foot in a patient with diabetes. The examiner uses the pointed end of a reflex hammer to strike the biceps, triceps, brachioradialis, patellar, and Achilles reflexes.

Tuning fork test

In this test, the examiner uses a tuning fork to assess peripheral nerve function and help identify and quantify existing neuropathy.

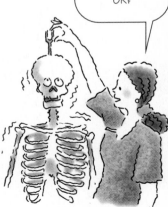

Just relax and focus on good vibrations, OK?

Name that tune

- The examiner activates the tuning fork and holds it against a bony prominence in the affected limb (for example, a metatarsal head or malleoli) and then records the patient's ability to sense the vibration.
- Next, the examiner tests other bony prominences in the body (for example, the patella or elbow) or the same prominence in the opposite limb if it's unaffected.
- Afterward, the results are compared to assess neurologic function.

Biothesiometer

A biothesiometer is another tool that's used to assess the patient's vibratory perception threshold. It provides a better quantitative measurement of vibratory sense than the tuning fork. Patients with sensory neuropathy have impaired vibratory perception thresholds (less than 25 volts, as measured on the biothesiometer).

Semmes-Weinstein test

The Semmes-Weinstein test helps determine the level of protective sensation in the feet. While the patient's eyes are closed, the examiner holds the Semmes-Weinstein monofilament perpendicular to the patient's foot and then presses the monofilament against the skin until it bows. The patient is then asked to identify when and where the skin has been touched. As protective sensation decreases, plantar pressures tend to rise, as does the patient's risk of ulcers at these points. (See *Performing the Semmes-Weinstein test.*)

Vascular tests

Vascular tests help assess circulation in the lower extremities. These tests include pulse palpation, ABI, measuring toe pressures, and obtaining transcutaneous oxygen (TcPO$_2$) levels.

Pulse palpation

Initial assessment of limb perfusion includes palpating the dorsalis pedis, posterior tibial, popliteal, and femoral pulses. If it's hard to palpate a pulse due to edema, consider using Doppler ultrasound, which produces an audible signal coinciding with the pulse.

Hear the beat

Hold the transducer at a 45-degree angle to the skin and listen for the beats. The results provide a general idea of the circulation to each level of the limb. A palpable dorsalis pedis pulse is roughly

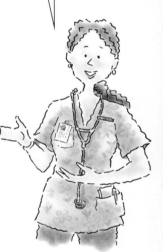

When performing the Semmes-Weinstein test, you'll use a monofilament to test the patient's level of protective sensation in his feet.

Performing the Semmes-Weinstein test

In the Semmes-Weinstein test, the examiner uses a special monofilament to assess protective sensation in the patient's feet. This illustration shows the points to test.

How it's done

The examiner places the 10-g monofilament on one of the testing points and exerts enough pressure to bow the monofilament (as illustrated). With his eyes closed, the patient must then identify where and when he feels the monofilament touch.

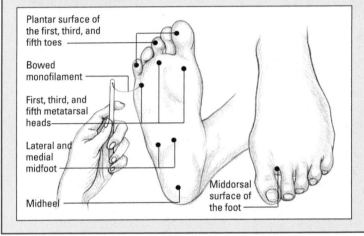

Plantar surface of the first, third, and fifth toes

Bowed monofilament

First, third, and fifth metatarsal heads

Lateral and medial midfoot

Midheel

Middorsal surface of the foot

equivalent to 80 mm Hg, which is adequate for healing most diabetic wounds. (See *Pulse rating,* page 174.)

Ankle-brachial index

PVD and resulting poor perfusion are common problems for patients with diabetes. Poor perfusion increases the patient's likelihood of developing ulcers and reduces the speed with which existing ulcers heal. Although this test is less reliable in a patient with diabetes, ABI is used in conjunction with other vascular tests to determine and monitor the patient's risk of ischemia in the area of the ankle. ABI is a ratio of systolic blood pressure in the brachial artery in the arm to systolic blood pressure measured in the dorsalis pedis artery in the ankle. However, the ABI may not be accurate in patients with diabetes if the vessels being measured are calcified and, therefore, not compressible. A falsely high reading may be seen due to incompressible artery walls caused by medial sclerosis of the arteries. (For more information on ABI, see chapter 6, Pressure ulcers.)

Pulse rating

When assessing the amplitude of a pulse, rate the strength on a numeric scale, such as the one below.

Rating	Pulse characteristic
0	No palpable pulse
+1	Weak or thready pulse: hard to feel, easily obliterated by slight finger pressure
+2	Normal pulse: easily palpable, obliterated by strong finger pressure
+3	Bounding pulse: readily palpable, forceful, not easily obliterated by finger pressure

Toe pressures

Toe pressures may be a more sensitive indicator of changes in vascular integrity in the distal areas of the foot. Toe pressures are performed in the same manner as limb blood pressures, except that a much smaller, specialized cuff is used for the toe. Due to the tiny arteries in digits, the corresponding arterial pressures are lower than those measured in an arm or a leg. Typical pressure in the toe is about 70% of systolic values obtained in the arm.

What the toes know

A toe pressure of 45 mm Hg or higher is needed for healing to occur. Toe pressures allow you to gauge the patient's ischemic risk profile. Generally, a toe pressure:
- above 55 mm Hg reflects a low risk of tissue ischemia
- below 40 mm Hg reflects a high risk of ischemia
- below 20 mm Hg reflects a severe risk of ischemia.

Transcutaneous oxygen levels

A $TcPO_2$ of 30% or higher is required for healing. $TcPO_2$ levels reflect the oxygen saturation of tissues. Typically, $TcPO_2$ levels are measured close to the ulcer. In general, a $TcPO_2$ level:
- above 40% reflects a low risk of tissue ischemia
- between 20% and 30% reflects a high risk of ischemia
- below 20% reflects a severe risk of ischemia.

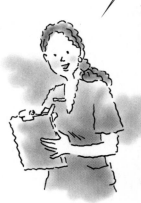

Your patient needs a toe pressure of 45 mm Hg or higher in order to heal.

Classification

Diabetic foot ulcers are classified according to depth, presence of ischemia, and presence of infection, depending on the classification system. The Wagner Ulcer Grade Classification and the University of Texas Diabetic Foot Classification System are two commonly used classification systems.

Wagner Ulcer Grade Classification

The original Wagner Ulcer Grade Classification considers depth of penetration; however, it doesn't allow for the assessment of infection at all tissue levels. A modified version of the Wagner classification system adds levels to take into account infection and ischemia. (See *Wagner Ulcer Grade Classification.*)

Wagner Ulcer Grade Classification

In the Wagner Ulcer Grade Classification, less complex ulcers receive lower scores; more complex ulcers, higher scores. Ulcers with higher scores may require surgical intervention or amputation.

Grade	Characteristics
0	• Preulcer lesion • Healed ulcer • Presence of bony deformity
1	• Superficial ulcer without subcutaneous tissue involvement
2	• Penetration through the subcutaneous tissue; may expose bone, tendon, ligament, or joint capsule
3	• Osteitis, abscess, or osteomyelitis
4	• Gangrene of a digit
5	• Gangrene requiring foot amputation

Adapted with permission from Wagner, F.W., Jr. "The Diabetic Foot," *Orthopedics* 10:163-72, 1987. © Slack Incorporated.

University of Texas Diabetic Foot Classification System

The University of Texas classification system takes tissue infection and ischemia into consideration and provides a more detailed breakdown of classifications than the Wagner system. (See *University of Texas Diabetic Foot Classification System.*)

Complications

The most common complication that impedes the healing of diabetic foot ulcers and can cause a wound to become chronic is infection. Other complications include:
• multiple comorbidities, including PVD, which cause a number of problems that increase the risk of ulceration and reduce the likelihood of speedy healing
• uncontrolled hyperglycemia, which commonly signals infection and inhibits the immune system, particularly the scavenging function of neutrophils
• psychosocial problems, such as depression and poverty, which profoundly affect the patient's nutritional status, in turn affecting the body's ability to prevent ulcers and heal existing wounds.

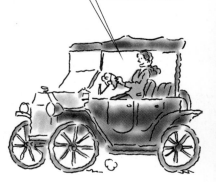

Comorbidities are speed bumps on the remedial road. They can slow healing of existing ulcers and contribute to new ones.

University of Texas Diabetic Foot Classification System

The University of Texas Diabetic Foot Classification System provides a detailed categorization of diabetic foot ulcers. Staging the ulcer from A to D is a predictor of amputation (stage D is at greatest risk) and grading it from 0 to III is an indicator of infection (grade III is at greatest risk).

Stage	Grade 0	Grade I	Grade II	Grade III
A	Preulcerative or postulcerative foot at risk for further ulceration	Superficial ulcer without tendon, capsule, or bone involvement	Ulcer penetrating to tendon or joint capsule	Ulcer penetrating to bone
B	Presence of infection	Presence of infection	Presence of infection	Presence of infection
C	Presence of ischemia	Presence of ischemia	Presence of ischemia	Presence of ischemia
D	Presence of infection and ischemia	Presence of infection and ischemia	Presence of infection and ischemia	Presence of infection and ischemia

Adapted with permission from Armstrong, D.G., et al. "Treatment-based Classification System for Assessment and Care of Diabetic Feet," *JAPMA* 86(7):311-16, July 1996.

Infection

An infection in the wound or elsewhere consumes protein needed for healing and interferes directly by damaging the wound bed. Infections fall into two categories: non-limb-threatening or limb-threatening. Non-limb-threatening infections tend to be superficial infections involving tissues within 2 cm of the wound margin. In this type of infection, no significant tissue ischemia is present and bone isn't palpable in the wound bed. Non-limb-threatening infection can be treated with topical antimicrobials, sharp debridement, and wound cleaning once or twice daily.

In contrast, limb-threatening infection involves tissue more than 2 cm from the wound margin, palpable bone in the wound bed, and tissue ischemia. When this occurs, hospitalization and surgical debridement of infected bone and soft tissues is necessary. Unless the infected bone is fully resected, the patient requires 4 to 8 weeks of I.V. antibiotic therapy.

Show me a sign

Uncontrollable blood glucose or hyperglycemia may be the first sign of infection because patients with diabetes commonly fail to demonstrate the typical systemic responses. A 4° to 5° difference in temperature between similar areas on each foot is a local sign of infection. An infrared scanner thermometer is the most reliable way to check this difference. An infection in the wound bed commonly causes friable (easy to bleed), bright-red granulation tissue.

Oste-oh-my-elitis

Osteomyelitis or bone infection is common in deep wounds. A quick and reliable method for determining whether osteomyelitis is present in a diabetic ulcer bed is to palpate for bone. A palpable bone usually indicates osteomyelitis; however, osteomyelitis may be difficult to distinguish from acute Charcot's neuropathic osteoarthropathy. The best way to differentiate between the two is to culture a bone fragment from the wound bed.

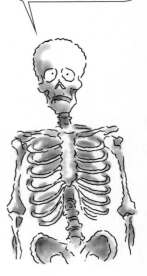

If you palpate bone in a diabetic ulcer bed, your patient probably has osteomyelitis. Culture a bone fragment to make sure. No ifs, ands, or bones about it!

Treatment

Successful healing depends on proper wound cleaning and dressing and off-loading. Topical antimicrobials, debridement, biotherapies, and surgery may also be included in the care plan.

Wound cleaning

Wound cleaning is a fundamental step in the healing process because necrotic tissue is a reservoir for bacteria and inhibits wound healing.

Flushing the wound bed with normal saline solution is the best method of cleaning a diabetic foot ulcer. Most commercial wound cleaners are somewhat toxic to cells in the wound bed; thus, their use can slow healing. Use clean, warm water and mild soap to clean the surrounding skin.

Helping hands

Cleaning the wound bed can be made easier by using bulb syringes, syringes with angiocatheters, aerosolized saline in a canister, pulsatile lavage with suction, and whirlpool. (For more information on wound cleaning, see chapter 3, Basic wound care procedures.)

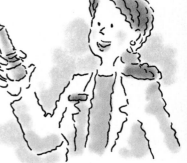

Devices, such as bulb syringes and syringes with angiocatheters, can help make cleaning the wound bed easier.

Dressings

Moist wound therapy speeds healing in diabetic foot ulcers. Dressings that maintain the necessary wound environment include:
- alginates
- transparent films
- foams
- hydrocolloids
- hydrogels
- collagen-based dressings
- composites (combinations of the other dressings)
- antimicrobials
- hydrofibers
- silver-impregnated dressings.

Choose wisely, my son

The dressing you choose depends on the condition of your patient's ulcer. Diabetic foot ulcers tend to produce low to moderate drainage; however, if the wound bed is dry, it needs a dressing that adds moisture. Either amorphous hydrogels or sheet hydrogels can help in this case. Hydrogel sheets are more cost-effective but don't work as well in deeper wounds. For deep or tunneling ulcers that require packing, hydrogel-impregnated gauze is an excellent, less costly alternative to amorphous hydrogels. All hydrogel dressings add moisture to the wound bed because they're made up of as much as 95% water. Hydrogels also encourage autolytic debridement. (See *Dressings for diabetic foot ulcers*.)

Dress for success

Dressings for diabetic foot ulcers

Use this chart to help you choose an appropriate dressing for your patient's foot ulcer.

Type of ulcer	Recommended dressings
Dry	• Hydrogel
Wet	• Alginate • Foam • Collagen
Necrotic	• Hydrogel • Hydrocolloid
Shallow	• Transparent film • Hydrocolloid
Tunneling or deep	• Alginate ropes (for wet ulcers) • Hydrogel-impregnated gauze (for dry ulcers)
Infected	• Iodosorb (a gel that cleans the wound by absorbing fluid, exudate, and bacteria) • Acticoat or Arglaes (products with an antimicrobial component)
Bleeding	• Alginate

Off-loading

Off-loading (relieving pressure) plantar tissues is the cornerstone of diabetic neuropathy treatment as well as prevention for those patients at risk for recurrent breakdown. Off-loading seeks to control, limit, or remove all intrinsic and extrinsic factors that increase plantar pressures. Examples of intrinsic risk factors include faulty biomechanics in the foot or the presence of a bony deformity. Extrinsic risk factors include trauma, ill-fitting shoes, or maintaining a position for too long, which allows for the buildup of damaging pressure.

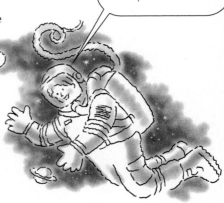

Relieving pressure from plantar surfaces — known as off-loading — is key to pressure ulcer treatment and prevention.

Damage control

Because patients with diabetic neuropathy can no longer feel the growing discomfort that precedes tissue damage, off-loading is particularly important. Both nonsurgical and surgical off-loading interventions help prevent or limit the kind of tissue damage that causes ulcers to form.

Nonsurgical off-loading interventions

Nonsurgical interventions include therapeutic footwear, custom orthotics, and walking casts. When considering a device, keep in mind that using a device can increase the patient's risk of falling. Be sure to provide instructions on fall prevention.

Therapeutic footwear

A patient with recurring ulcers and severe foot deformities can greatly benefit from a custom-molded shoe. Common design features of therapeutic footwear include:
• soft, breathable leather that conforms to foot deformities
• high tops for ankle stability
• rocker soles and bottoms for pressure and pain relief across the plantar metatarsal heads
• a toe box with extra depth and width to accommodate deformities, such as clawed toes and hallux valgus (displacement of the great toe toward the other toes)
• flared lateral soles for stability. (See *Therapeutic shoe modifications.*)

Custom orthotics

Custom orthotics are shoe inserts that serve various functions based on the patient's needs. In general, custom orthotics relieve pressure, reduce shearing force and friction, and cushion the foot against shocks. If necessary, custom orthotics accommodate the patient's foot deformities as well.

Walking casts

Walking casts range from total contact casts to splints and walkers.

Cast member

A total contact cast is the top of the line in care for uninfected diabetic ulcers on the plantar surface of the foot. Total contact casts are custom made for each patient by a health care professional, typically a physical therapist or orthotist. Inside the cast, padding is fitted over bony areas of the ankle and leg that are at risk for pressure ulcers. A plaster shell reinforced with plaster splints covers the padding. Fiberglass covers the plaster to lend rigidity and additional

Therapeutic shoe modifications

These illustrations show the modifications in custom shoes that can improve stability and accommodate the deformities that affect many patients with diabetes.

High top

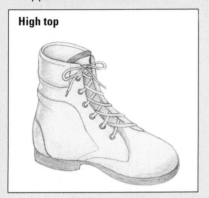

Lateral flare

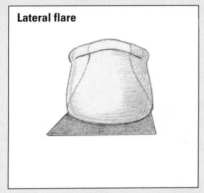

Rocker sole

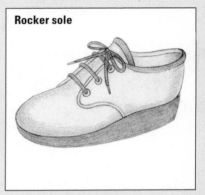

strength, and the cast includes a sturdy walking heel for ambulation. The cast is molded to fit snugly to prevent the foot from sliding inside it. This reduces shearing forces over the plantar surface.

A patient with an infected diabetic ulcer isn't a candidate for a total contact cast because a cast makes daily assessment, cleaning, and antimicrobial therapy impossible. In addition, inflammation and edema can cause a buildup of pressure within the cast and subsequent tissue damage. In the case of infection, a removable off-loading device should be used.

Walk this way

Splints and walkers have cushioned inserts with an outer shell of fiberglass or copolymer. Several splint and walker options are available. One advantage of splints and walkers is that they allow easy inspection of the ulcer. In addition, off-loading modifications can be accomplished relatively easily by changing the type of splint or walker in use. However, these devices have disadvantages as well. First and foremost, they don't provide the same degree of pressure and shear relief as a total contact cast. Also, for these therapies to work, the patient must be committed to using the device—a patient can always take a splint off or choose not to use a walker.

Surgical off-loading interventions

Surgical off-loading procedures include surgical dissection of the wound bed and pressure-inducing bony tissue deformities. Pres-

A total contact cast is out of the question for a patient with an infected foot ulcer. Instead, use a removable off-loading device.

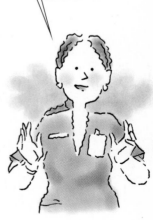

sure over bony prominences compresses and occludes blood vessels, causing ischemia. Resection (surgical removal) of bony deformities reduces peak plantar pressures. This type of surgery is called *curative surgery* because it removes the pathologic tissue. Examples of curative surgery include exostectomy, digital arthroplasty, bone and joint resections, and partial calcanectomy.

Topical antimicrobials

Routine wound cleaning handles much of the surface microbial population; however, applying a topical antimicrobial directly to the wound bed can help control microorganisms in the wound bed and improve healing. Commonly used topical antimicrobials include:

- bacitracin (Baciguent)
- metronidazole (MetroGel)
- mupirocin (Bactroban)
- silver sulfadiazine (Silvadene).

Keep in mind that some microorganisms are resistant to certain topical agents. In addition, recent findings indicate that neomycin-containing products (such as Neosporin) can cause allergic reactions. Consequently, these are no longer recommended for ulcer treatment.

The next generation

Newer wound care antimicrobials include Iodosorb gel, Iodoflex pad, Arglaes antimicrobial barrier, and Acticoat. These products contain iodine or silver, which kills or inhibits microbes. The active ingredients are released slowly in concentrations that are toxic to microbes but not to important cells in the wound bed such as fibroblasts. As an added benefit, research seems to indicate that microbes aren't as likely to develop resistance to this new generation of products.

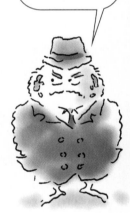

Foiled again! Using a topical antimicrobial on the wound bed helps keep out microorganisms like me. That improves healing!

Debridement

Debriding necrotic and nonviable tissue, foreign matter, and microbes from the wound bed expedites wound healing. The most effective method of debridement, surgical debridement is required in cases of osteomyelitis or when the wound involves a deep abscess or spreading tissue infection. Sharp debridement, which can be performed at the bedside, is an option when surgery isn't necessary or the patient is a poor surgical candidate. Topical proteolytic enzymes can be applied to wound tissue to augment debridement between sessions. (For more information on wound debridement, see chapter 3, Basic wound care procedures.)

Biotherapies

Growth factors and living skin equivalents are two forms of biotherapy that may be included in the care plan for a patient with a diabetic foot ulcer.

Growth factors

Growth factors orchestrate healing in the wound bed. One factor in particular — platelet-derived growth factor (PDGF) — is called the *master factor*. PDGF plays a central role by stimulating chemotaxis and the proliferation of neutrophils, fibroblasts, and monocytes. In clinical trials, the PDGF-based product becaplermin (Regranex gel 0.01%) increased wound closure rates. However, this therapy also relies on an adequate vascular supply, proper wound bed preparation, and glycemic control.

Living skin equivalents

Living skin equivalents are products composed of living cells and a matrix, or scaffolding, that serves as the extracellular medium. These products act as interactive wound coverings, providing growth factors and other needed molecules. Dermagraft is one example of a living skin equivalent. It has viable fibroblasts that enhance wound healing rates in diabetic ulcers. Graftskin (Apligraf), another living skin equivalent, also accelerates wound healing.

> Living skin equivalents, such as Dermagraft and Apligraf, contribute viable fibroblasts that enhance diabetic ulcer healing.

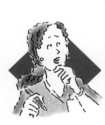

Quick quiz

1. The single greatest risk factor for diabetic foot ulcers is:
   A. PVD.
   B. peripheral neuropathy.
   C. retinitis pigmentosa.
   D. myopathy.

   Answer: B. Peripheral neuropathy is the primary risk factor for diabetic foot ulcers.

2. Diabetic ulceration can commonly be found:
   A. around the ankle.
   B. over the sacrum.
   C. on the dorsal surface of the foot.
   D. on the plantar surface of the foot.

Answer: D. Always check the plantar surfaces of the feet for signs of ulcerations. Also check between toes and on the tips of toes.

3. Which complication commonly results from motor neuropathy?
  A. Charcot's neuropathic osteoarthropathy
  B. Diminished sensation
  C. Clawed toes
  D. Poor circulation

Answer: C. Clawed toes commonly result from motor neuropathy, a long-term complication of diabetes.

4. The Semmes-Weinstein test is used to assess:
  A. blood flow to the feet.
  B. protective sensation of the feet.
  C. pressure on the feet.
  D. temperature of the feet.

Answer: B. During the Semmes-Weinstein test, the examiner uses a monofilament to assess the patient's protective sensation, or the ability to detect stimuli that may be harmful to the feet.

5. Which statement about the total contact cast is true?
  A. It's a method of relieving pressure on the foot.
  B. It's a special cast for fractures due to Charcot's neuropathic osteoarthropathy.
  C. It's recommended for use over infected diabetic foot ulcerations.
  D. It's removable.

Answer: A. The total contact cast is an off-loading device that relieves pressure on the foot. However, because it isn't removable, it isn't recommended for use over infected wounds.

Scoring

☆☆☆ If you answered all five questions correctly, you've got a reason to grin! You off-loaded this quiz in a jiffy.

☆☆ If you answered four questions correctly, brag to your friends! You zipped through this quiz with no friction or shear.

☆ If you answered fewer than four questions correctly, let out a sigh! Plantar your feet and move onward and upward.

8

Nonhealing wounds

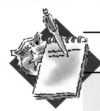

Just the facts

In this chapter, you'll learn:

♦ causes of nonhealing wounds

♦ assessment of nonhealing wounds

♦ management of nonhealing wounds

♦ important teaching points for patients and their caregivers.

A look at nonhealing wounds

A nonhealing wound is typically defined as a wound that fails to follow the normal healing process. When all standard approaches to wound healing fail, the wound becomes chronic and is classified as nonhealing.

Factors that affect healing

Nonhealing wounds are a distressing problem for patients, their caregivers, and the health care community. Socioeconomic and psychological factors commonly play a role in determining whether a wound will heal.

Socioeconomic factors

Socioeconomic factors can play an important role in determining the patient's ability to comply with a treatment plan. The patient on a fixed income may not be able to afford to make the choice between wound treatment, housing, and food. If you have a patient who's in this situation, consult social services to determine if alternative payment sources can be found. In time, you may also need to make changes to the treatment plan in order to decrease the patient's costs. Remember to periodically assess the patient for changes in status.

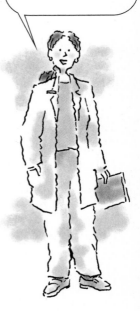

When all standard approaches to wound healing fail, the wound becomes chronic and is classified as nonhealing.

Money matters

Income can impact the patient's living conditions as well. Poor living conditions can influence his ability to heal. It's important to evaluate the patient's home environment and assess its condition and the ability of the patient and his family to manage the wound within that environment. A referral to home health care may be appropriate to assist the patient and his family with wound management.

Working for the man

In addition, the patient's work history can influence his risk for development of cancer and malignant wounds. Job loss due to this health crisis can also leave him without health insurance coverage. A patient who doesn't have adequate insurance may be unable to purchase necessary wound care supplies or seek appropriate follow-up care. In an older patient with a nonhealing wound, Medicare may not cover all the necessary required treatments, leaving the patient to pay a portion of the costs, which he may be unable to do.

Take attendance

The patient's education level is also an important factor in nonhealing wound management. Because the care of these wounds is complicated, you need to consider the patient's education level to ensure that he's able to understand how to manage his wound. You may need to alter your teaching regarding the wound and its treatment plan so that the patient and his family can understand your instructions.

Cultural cues

Cultural or religious beliefs may prevent the patient from seeking appropriate medical attention or complying with the wound treatment plan. In order to improve the patient's compliance with the plan, evaluate his cultural and religious beliefs to ensure that the treatment plan is in accordance with them.

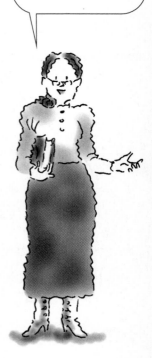

Consider your patient's education level when teaching him how to care for his nonhealing wound.

Psychological factors

Excessive wound exudate, bleeding, and odor may lead the patient to isolate himself from his family and social situations rather than risk embarrassment. In addition, feelings of embarrassment can cause the patient to feel less attractive to his partner. For this reason, you should assess the patient for changes in sexuality. Also, many partners become caregivers, performing wound care and hygiene for the patient. This may cause the relationship between the patient and his partner to become more like a patient-caregiver relationship rather than an intimate one. Such issues can lead to depression. Be sure to provide opportunities for the patient and his caregivers to discuss their concerns. Support groups may also become an important source of support and nurturing.

Causes

The two most common causes of nonhealing wounds are infection and malignancy. Nonhealing wounds can also be caused by inadequate perfusion resulting from chronic disease.

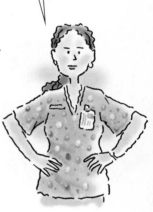

Infection, malignancy, and inadequate perfusion can cause nonhealing wounds.

Infection

Studies suggest that infection may account for about 40% of nonhealing wounds. Nonhealing wounds may be infected with *Klebsiella*, *Proteus*, *Pseudomonas*, *Staphylococcus*, *Clostridium*, and *Bacteroides fragilis*. Typically, these infected wounds don't show any classic signs of infection, such as edema, redness, and purulent drainage. In some instances, prolonged inflammation longer than 5 days; discolored or bleeding, friable granulation tissue; pocketing at the base of the wound; and the absence of healing may be the only signs of infection.

Detective work

If an infection remains undetected, the wound won't heal. This can lead to amputations and other serious complications such as osteomyelitis. When a wound fails to heal, suspect infection and evaluate the wound accordingly.

Malignancy

Patients can also develop nonhealing wounds as a result of a malignancy. About 6% to 10% of cancer patients develop nonhealing, malignant wounds. Some cancers may ulcerate as they outgrow their blood supply, and some chronic wounds have been known to develop into squamous cell carcinomas. A nonhealing, malignant wound may appear at the site of malignant disease or at a site distal to the malignancy. These types of wounds are most commonly associated with breast cancer but they can also occur from other malignancies, such as cancer of the head, neck, chest, abdomen, kidney, lung, ovary, colon and penis as well as from leukemia, lymphoma, and melanoma.

Disorganization dilemma

Cancer cells are typically disorganized with poorly differentiated borders as a result of the malignant change that alters their normal behavior. When a cell becomes cancerous, it begins to rob surrounding tissues of oxygen and nutrients. Malignant cells begin to secrete tissue permeability factor, which increases vascular permeability. This leads to increased production of exudates, which causes loss of protein and fibrinogen. Thus, malignant wounds are prone to bleeding because they're highly vascular and have poor clotting tendencies.

Breaking down

Bacterial proteases (enzymes present in necrotic tissue) cause the breakdown of tissue. Malignant wounds tend to have a large amount of necrotic tissue because they fail to heal; therefore, they also have an increased number of bacterial proteases present. With the presence of nonviable, necrotic tissue and excessive drainage, malignant wounds provide an ideal medium for aerobic and anaerobic organism growth, which can cause these wounds to have a foul odor. Aerobic bacteria that may cause odor include *Klebsiella*, *Proteus*, *Pseudomonas*, and *Staphylococcus*. Anaerobic bacteria that may cause odor include *Clostridium* and *Bacteroides fragilis*.

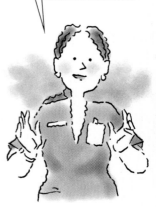

Aerobic and anaerobic organisms commonly grow in malignant wounds, causing a foul odor.

Size reducers

Chemotherapy and radiation treatments can reduce the size of a malignant wound. The smaller wound may become more manageable in terms of drainage, odor, and bleeding. However, chemotherapy and radiation may also cause periwound (skin around the wound) irritation, which may lead to further wound development.

A slow leak

Wounds can also develop if chemotherapy drugs leak into the tissues. In addition, some cytoxic drugs are irritants and will cause pain or inflammation without necrosis, while other drugs, known as *vesicants*, can cause severe pain and may result in severe tissue damage.

Radiation-induced skin damage can appear in different ways:
- mild erythema and edema similar to a sunburn
- dry desquamation characterized by hyperpigmented, intact skin that's dry, itching, peeling, and flaking
- moist desquamation or partial-thickness injury with blistering
- deep dermal damage to hair follicles and sweat or sebaceous glands
- ulcerations and necrosis.

Additionally, radiation recall can occur in the field of treatment when chemotherapy is given concurrently or subsequent to radiation therapy with skin damage that occurs several weeks after the radiation has ended.

Chronic diseases

Nonhealing wounds may also develop as a result of inadequate tissue perfusion caused by such chronic diseases as diabetes, chronic obstructive pulmonary disease, vascular insufficiency, and anemia. These disorders can also increase the patient's risk of developing infections in an open wound, especially anaerobic infections.

Assessment

When you assess a patient for a nonhealing wound, obtain a thorough patient history and perform a physical examination.

History

If you suspect a nonhealing wound, you need to gather information about the wound's development. Remember to ask the patient these questions:
• When did the wound develop?
• What past or current wound treatments have you undergone (if any)? When was your last chemotherapy or radiation treatment (if applicable)?
• Has the appearance of the wound changed?
• Is there drainage from the wound? If so, what's the color and odor of the drainage?

  Then assess the patient's medication history, the presence of diseases, and his nutritional status.

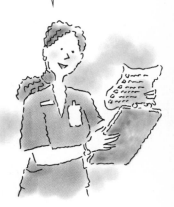

When obtaining a patient history, be sure to ask the patient when his wound developed and ask about any past or current treatments, including medications he may be taking.

Medications

Certain medications may influence wound healing. Keep in mind that such medications as steroids, antivirals, antibiotics, and antineoplastics can be immunosuppressive, affecting the body's ability to respond to a wound infection. Herbal and other nontraditional medications can also influence the patient's risk for infection. When you obtain a medication history, remember to ask if the patient has used or is using any nontraditional medications.

Diseases

The presence of more than one disease may also increase the patient's risk for infection. Ask the patient about a history of diseases that impact the vascular, pulmonary, and immune systems.

Diseases, such as cancer, autoimmune disorders, and acquired immunodeficiency syndrome, can impact the body's ability to respond to infection and can alter the appearance of an infected wound. If the patient's immune system is compromised, an infected wound may fail to exhibit the traditional symptoms of infection.

Cancer connection

Question the patient about a history of cancer, including the type of cancer and any metastasis to other sites. Remember that certain cancers are more likely to cause nonhealing wounds. Cancers of the head, neck, chest, and abdomen are the most common sites for malignant wounds.

Radiation ramifications

Treatment for cancer usually includes chemotherapy and radiation. Chemotherapy drugs can cause such adverse effects as immunosuppression, GI disturbances, and mucous membrane ulceration. GI disturbances, such as chronic diarrhea, can lead to excoriated skin, which can predispose the patient to infection and wound development. Immunosuppression can affect the body's ability to fight infection. In turn, ulceration of mucous membranes may cause wound development in an immunocompromised patient. Ask the patient when he last received chemotherapy and if he experienced adverse effects.

Radiation therapy can also contribute to the development of nonhealing wounds. If the patient is undergoing radiation treatment, determine the type of radiation and how many treatments have been administered and identify adverse effects the patient has experienced.

Nutritional status

The patient's nutritional status can influence the development of a nonhealing wound and whether it will eventually heal. Evaluate the patient's diet to determine if he's consuming enough calories and protein to promote wound healing. Obtaining blood tests, such as albumin, pre-albumin, and electrolyte levels, can also provide important information about the patient's nutritional status.

If you discover that the patient is malnourished, try to find the cause. The patient may fail to consume enough calories for various reasons, including lack of money, disliking the taste of the food, or poor appetite. All of these factors must be considered when discussing a nutritional plan

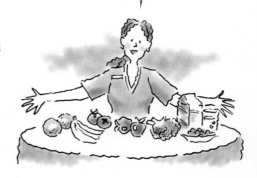

Poor nutrition can influence the development of a nonhealing wound. Be sure to evaluate your patient's diet to determine if he's consuming enough calories and protein.

with the patient. Keep in mind that cultural influences can also impact compliance with an ordered diet.

Mom always says, take your vitamins...

Remember, the patient with a nonhealing wound needs to increase his consumption of protein and his caloric intake because a nonhealing wound tends to have excessive exudate, which leads to a loss of protein. In addition, encourage the patient to take multivitamins to ensure that he's getting an adequate amount of vitamins and minerals.

...And eat your veggies

Vegetable protein powder sprinkled into food and drinks can increase the protein content in the patient's diet without affecting the taste of the food. Protein shakes and bars are also good options for increasing protein in the diet.

He's got no taste

Keep in mind that chemotherapy and radiation can alter a patient's sense of taste. For example, some chemotherapeutic drugs will cause a metallic taste in the mouth. The GI disturbances commonly caused by chemotherapy and radiation, such as nausea, vomiting, and ulcerations, can lower a patient's tolerance for foods. In addition, the psychological effects of a life-threatening illness coupled with a nonhealing wound can cause anorexia and malnourishment.

> We proteins really deliver when patients with nonhealing wounds lose too much of us due to excessive exudate.

Physical examination

Assess a wound that fails to follow the normal healing process for infection. The wound may have nonviable or hypertrophic tissue and may demonstrate delays in epithelial migration leading to wound closure. Remember, in addition to assessing the wound, you should always perform a thorough physical examination, including vital signs. To determine the presence of an infection, evaluate the patient's wound for evidence of local and systemic infection and bone involvement.

Evidence of infection

Some wounds may demonstrate clear signs of infection, including erythema, edema, purulent drainage, unexpected or increased pain, and foul odor. Systemic signs of infection include cellulitis extending at least 1 cm beyond the wound margin, fever, elevated white blood cell (WBC) count, and a suddenly high blood glucose level. However, some wounds may fail to demonstrate the obvious signs of infection; therefore, you must carefully investigate the wound in order to determine if it's a nonhealing wound.

Behind the mask

Signs of infection in patients with diabetes or arterial disease may be subtle or masked. A wound that fails to follow the normal healing process should be assessed for infection. In some cases, inflammation that persists longer than 5 days; discolored or bleeding, friable granulation tissue; the presence of pocketing at the base of the wound; and the absence of healing may indicate infection.

A fungus among us

The first step is to examine the wound's appearance. Malignant wounds have been described as rapidly growing (like a fungus) and cauliflower-like in appearance. You may also find that the patient's wound has nonviable tissue and may bleed easily because malignant wounds tend to have poor perfusion and clotting tendencies. Carefully assess the malignant wound for the presence of sinus tracts or fistulas because malignant cells tend to invade surrounding tissues and organs.

As malignant cells invade the surrounding tissue, pruritus (itching) may develop due to stretching of the skin and irritation of peripheral nerve fibers. Fungal infections may also cause pruritus. Evaluate for pruritus and be sure to ask the patient about products he's using to alleviate the itching. Antihistamines typically have no effect on the pruritus that's associated with malignant wounds.

Color, consistency, and odor, oh my!

Malignant wounds may have copious amounts of exudate. These wounds may also have a foul odor. Assess the color, consistency, odor, and amount of wound exudate. You should also evaluate the periwound for maceration caused by exudate.

Bone involvement

An X-ray of the affected area can't be relied on to help determine bone involvement because it can take 10 to 21 days for bone changes to be visible on an X-ray. A bone biopsy is considered the gold standard when diagnosing osteomyelitis; however, because it's invasive, noninvasive tests, such as a bone scan or magnetic resonance imaging (MRI), are preferred.

Suspect osteomyelitis in any nonhealing wound that probes to the bone. Osteomyelitis is a serious complication in which bacterial organisms have invaded the bone tissue. It commonly leads to amputation of the affected extremity or removal of the infected bone.

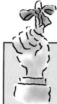

Memory jogger

Use the acronym **APEEP** to help you remember how to assess nonhealing wounds:

Assessment of the wound bed

Pain

Exudate

Emotional distress

Pruritus.

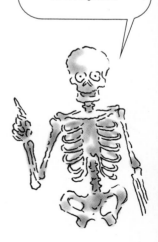

Noninvasive tests, such as a bone scan or MRI, are preferred when diagnosing osteomyelitis.

Diagnostic tests

Diagnostic tests that can be performed to determine if a wound is nonhealing include:
• WBC and differential count—used to obtain information about the presence and type of infection and whether the infection is acute or chronic (It can also help evaluate a client's immune system function which, if compromised, can lead to an increased risk for bleeding and poor tissue perfusion.)
• red blood cell and platelet count—used to evaluate the patient's immune function as a result of treatment with chemotherapy and radiation; a low count may indicate an increased risk for bleeding and poor tissue perfusion
• tissue biopsy—used to confirm the diagnosis of a malignant wound; particularly important if the wound developed without any known cause
• MRI and computed tomography and bone scans—used to obtain information regarding the metastasis of cancer and which organs and tissues the cancer has impacted (These tests also provide information about bone involvement and help diagnose osteomyelitis.)
• wound culture and sensitivity—used to determine the number and specific type of aerobic and anaerobic bacteria, which can also help determine appropriate antibiotic therapy.

Treatment

The primary purpose of any wound management system is to protect the wound and provide an ideal environment for wound healing. When treating nonhealing wounds, focus on controlling exudate, odor, and pain and be sure to select the proper dressing and therapeutic modality, depending on the patient's needs. With nonhealing wounds caused by a malignancy, the goals of treatment should be based on symptom control and comfort, rather than healing, at the end of life.

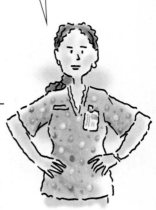

The goals of treating nonhealing, malignant wounds are symptom control and comfort.

Controlling exudate

Controlling exudate is one of the primary goals of nonhealing wound management. Several dressing options are available, including calcium alginate, foam, and hydrofiber dressings, which provide excellent absorption in wounds with moderate to large amounts of exudate. The use of wound drainage systems, such as pouches or suction systems, can also be a viable option for wounds with large amounts of exudate.

Calcium caution

Keep in mind that calcium alginate dressings may increase trauma to the wound bed and should be used with caution in bleeding wounds.

Controlling odor

Use dressings that contain charcoal, such as CarboFlex and Actisorb Plus, to control wound odor. Frequent dressing changes can also aid in odor control. In addition, the use of topical antibiotics may reduce bacterial load and reduce odor. The topical application of metronidazole (MetroGel) and the use of maltodextrin powder or gel have been reported to decrease and control odor in fungating wounds.

Controlling pain

Pain can be an important issue in nonhealing wounds. Be sure to assess the patient for pain by using a reliable and valid pain assessment tool, such as the visual analog, numeric pain intensity, or FACES pain rating scales, and make sure that appropriate pain management techniques are implemented. Premedication before dressing changes can increase the patient's comfort. Analgesics may be prescribed according to the World Health Organization's guidelines.

Topical solution

In addition, topical anesthetics may reduce the amount of pain experienced by the patient during dressing changes and throughout the day. Topical application of medications, such as EMLA cream, 30 to 60 minutes before debridement or dressing changes has been effective in reducing the pain associated with these procedures. Complementary therapies, such as massage, visualization, and aromatherapy, may also help the patient with pain control.

Dressings

In some nonhealing wounds, particularly malignant wounds, bleeding is an issue. Nonadherent dressings should be utilized to reduce trauma to the wound tissue and reduce the risk of bleeding. Contact layers made of soft silicone or petroleum-impregnated gauze will prevent outer dressings from sticking to the wound bed. Other appropriate dressings for a bleeding wound include foam, calcium alginate, and hydrofoam dressings. In addition, hemostatic dressings, such as calcium alginate, Spongostan, and Oxycel, encourage coagulation. (See *Dressings used for nonheal-*

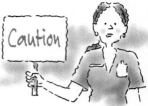

Be careful when using a calcium alginate dressing for a bleeding wound with minimal exudate because the dressing may adhere to the wound bed and damage tissue.

Caution

ing wounds.) Keep in mind that calcium alginate dressings are indicated for wounds with heavy drainage and should be used with caution in bleeding wounds with minimal exudate because they could adhere to the wound bed and damage tissue when removed.

Adrenaline rush

You may also use topical adrenaline, which causes local vasoconstriction and can assist in controlling bleeding. However, this vasoconstriction can lead to poor tissue perfusion, so remember to use with caution.

Debridement

Wound debridement and cleaning are effective measures to reduce the amount of nonviable tissue and the bacterial load in a

Dress for success

Dressings used for nonhealing wounds

Use this chart to help you determine which dressing or medication to use on a nonhealing wound.

Wound characteristics	Dressings	Medications
Exudate	• Foam • Calcium alginate • Hydrofiber • Sodium chloride-impregnated gauze	• Antibiotic creams
Odor	• Foam • Calcium alginate • Hydrofiber • Composite • Charcoal • Occlusive	• Topical metronidazole • Antibiotic creams
Pain	• Hydrogel (if wound has minimal drainage) • Foam • Calcium alginate • Hydrofiber • Nonadhesive	• Topical anesthetics • Oral or parenteral pain medications
Bleeding	• Foam • Hydrofiber • Hemostatic (such as Gelfoam, Spongostan, and Oxycel)	• Topical adrenaline (use with caution) • Silver nitrate (to cauterize bleeding)

wound. Several options are available, including autolysis; enzymatic, mechanical, surgical, or conservative sharp debridement; and biological (larvae) therapy.

The decision to use a specific method of debridement depends on several factors, such as:

- cause or source of the wound
- extent of infection
- amount and extent of necrosis
- type of tissue
- healing potential
- risk for bleeding and pain
- comorbidity factors
- the patient's and family's wishes.

Weighing the benefits

You should weigh the benefits of debridement against the risk of exposing the protected surface of a wound when healing may be delayed or isn't expected. In patients with nonhealing wounds related to poor tissue perfusion with no chance of tissue revascularization, debridement of the protective eschar can lead to further complications.

Antibiotics

Treat infection with antibiotics. Antibiotics may be applied topically to the wound bed or may be administered systemically. Perform a wound culture and sensitivity any time you suspect an infection to prevent complications and delays in wound healing. To perform an appropriate wound culture, flush the wound with normal saline solution or clean the wound with saline-moistened sterile gauze to remove surface contaminants. Then using sterile technique, swab the wound base with an alginate-tipped applicator over a 1 cm × 1 cm area for 5 seconds. Alternatively, you can rotate the applicator in a Z-track method (such as the 10-point technique). Remember to use sufficient pressure to express tissue fluid with either technique. (See *Performing a wound culture.*)

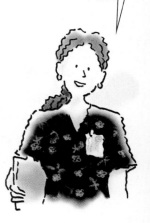

When educating the patient with a nonhealing wound, focus on symptom management.

Patient education

Focus on symptom management when educating a patient with a nonhealing wound. Instruct the patient and his caregivers about the correct procedure for dressing changes. Because pain management is an important issue affecting the patient's quality of life, you should instruct him in how to manage his pain effectively, including premedication before dressing changes. You should also include proper nutrition and odor control in the teaching plan.

Get wise to wounds

Performing a wound culture

A wound culture can be used to determine if a wound is infected. If the wound bed of a nonhealing wound is pink with viable tissue, a culture for aerobic organisms is indicated. However, you should perform a culture for both aerobic and anaerobic organisms in the presence of nonviable, necrotic tissue.

To perform an appropriate wound culture, follow these steps:

• First, flush the wound with normal saline solution.
• Then with a culture or calcium alginate swab, swab the wound using a 10-point technique.
• Go back and forth across the wound (as shown).

Remember, you don't want to culture eschar because the culture won't provide reliable results. If eschar is present, the wound should be debrided to allow for a culture, if appropriate.

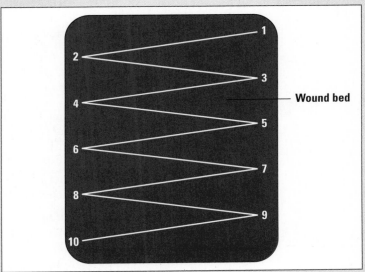

Wound bed

Strive for success

The success of any teaching plan relies heavily on the patient and his caregivers. Therefore, make sure the patient understands the plan and that it addresses any specific issues he may have. Remember that you'll need to periodically evaluate the effectiveness of your teaching plan and revise it based on your findings.

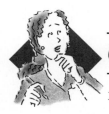

Quick quiz

1. You would suspect an infection in a nonhealing wound if:
    A. the wound bed is pink and granulation tissue is present.
    B. epithelial migration across the wound bed is delayed.
    C. small to moderate amounts of serous drainage are present.
    D. nonviable tissue is absent.

Answer: B. Epithelial migration is important in the normal wound healing process. A delay in epithelial migration indicates a potential infection.

2. You can prevent bleeding in a wound by:
A. applying wound gels.
B. using nonadherent dressings.
C. applying topical anesthetics.
D. using hydrocolloid dressings.

Answer: B. Nonadherent dressings reduce trauma to the wound bed and reduce bleeding.

3. The nurse is providing education to a group of patients with cancer about management of their nonhealing wounds. It's important for the nurse to:
A. review the patients' treatment plans.
B. consider individual wound management priorities.
C. verify the types of cancer.
D. determine the locations of the wounds.

Answer: B. The nurse must consider what issues are important to each patient in order to improve compliance.

4. A patient informs the nurse that he lost his job because of excessive absences related to his wound. The nurse would:
A. evaluate the patient's understanding of his wound management.
B. explain to the patient that he can no longer be seen at the clinic without a job.
C. encourage the patient to express his feelings about the job loss.
D. contact social services to assist the patient with accessing available resources.

Answer: D. Job loss and subsequent loss of insurance coverage can be an important factor in noncompliance with wound management, which can lead to delayed wound healing.

Scoring

⭐⭐⭐ If you answered all four questions correctly, give yourself a pat on the back! You've mastered the basics of nonhealing wounds.

⭐⭐ If you answered three questions correctly, it's a "non" issue! You're doing just fine.

⭐ If you answered fewer than three questions correctly, you aren't at risk! A quick review will heal your score in no time.

9

Wound care products

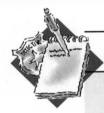

Just the facts

In this chapter, you'll learn:

♦ criteria to use when selecting wound care products

♦ types of dressings used in wound care and the characteristics, indications, advantages, and disadvantages of each type

♦ products that are used in conjunction with dressings, including their indications, advantages, and disadvantages.

A look at wound care products

Over time, wound care has developed from a practice that focused primarily on care of the injury to a process that also considers the complexities of the patient's general health, possible underlying disease, and specific wound characteristics. As wound care knowledge has increased, so have the number and types of products available to aid healing.

As you read, keep in mind that dressings and adjunct wound care products are tools that can help promote full healing, but they aren't the only tools you'll need. Unless concurrent problems, such as malnutrition, circulatory disorders, and patient knowledge deficits, are also addressed, the healing process stalls. In addition, no dressing or topical agent can compensate for an incomplete assessment. In short, let the findings of a thorough assessment guide your wound care product selection. (See *Tips for selecting wound care products*, page 200.)

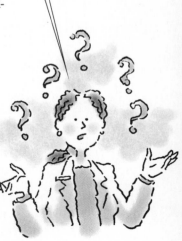

The abundance of commercially prepared dressings and adjunct products — and the fact that many have similar names and functions — can make choosing the right product a daunting task.

Tips for selecting wound care products

When selecting wound care products, let the big picture guide your choices. Ask yourself these important questions:
- Which companies have contracts to supply wound care products to your facility? (Learn about these products first.)
- What's the simplest method of closing the wound? Which is most cost-effective?
- Can the patient afford the supplies he needs? (Simple and affordable aren't necessarily synonymous.) If not, is financial assistance available?
- Who provides wound care at home? If the patient can't perform this important task, can family members or friends help? Is home health care an option? If so, is the patient eligible?
- What caused the wound and how can the cause best be alleviated? (This is especially important when treating chronic wounds; less so when treating acute wounds.)
- How often does the dressing need to be changed? (It usually takes at least 8 hours for a wound to achieve homeostasis after a dressing change. Therefore, the less often dressing changes are needed, the better.)
- How much drainage is present?
- Does the wound need more moisture?
- Should the wound be debrided? If so, which method is best for the patient?
- After cleaning and drying, does the wound (not the dressing) have an unpleasant odor? Do you suspect infection? If so, is a culture warranted?
- Is there tunneling, undermining, or a cavity that needs to be filled?
- Are the wound edges open or closed? (Wound edges must be open for complete healing to occur.)
- How large is the wound? Would it be more cost-effective to use an advanced wound care product to facilitate granulation tissue or closure?

All the rage

Keep in mind that new products arrive almost daily and others are updated or improved regularly. Because the quality of the care that you provide depends on your level of knowledge, it's imperative that you stay up-to-date by periodically reviewing the available products.

Wound dressings

Gauze has been a core wound dressing for more years than any other material. However, as medical research has afforded a better understanding of wounds and the healing process, manufacturers have developed new materials and sophisticated dressing options that promote better healing.

Moisture level, tissue adherence, infection control, and wound dimensions are just some of the factors that affect wound dressing selection. The level of moisture in the wound bed is critical to the success or failure of healing. Consequently, one fundamental way to classify dressings is by their effect on wound moisture. Ask yourself, does the dressing add, absorb, or not affect wound moisture? (See *Dressing for the occasion*.)

Dressing for the occasion

Some dressings absorb moisture from a wound bed; some add moisture to it. Others help maintain the existing moisture level. Use this chart to quickly determine the category of dressing that's appropriate for your patient.

MOISTURE SCALE

Absorb moisture		Neutral (maintain existing moisture level)		Add moisture	
• Alginates • Specialty absorptives • Vacuum-assisted Closure (VAC) devices • Gauze	• Foams • Hydrocolloids • Compression dressings	• Composites • VAC devices	• Transparent films • Biological dressings • Collagen dressings • Contact layers • Warm-Up Therapy System	• Sheet hydrogels	• Amorphous hydrogels • Debriding agents • Antimicrobial dressings

Gauze but not forgotten

Although gauze remains a good choice for secondary dressings, it no longer represents the most effective choice for a primary dressing. Other dressings you can use include alginate, antimicrobial, biological, collagen, composite, contact layer, foam, hydrocolloid, hydrogel, specialty absorbtive, and transparent film. Wound fillers are also available.

Alginate dressings

Made from seaweed, alginate dressings are nonwoven and absorptive. They're available as soft, white, sterile pads or ropes. Alginate dressings absorb excessive exudate and may be used on infected wounds. As they absorb exudate, they turn into a gel that keeps the wound bed moist and promotes healing. These nonadhesive and nonocclusive dressings also promote autolysis.

Examples of alginate dressings include:
- AlgiSite M
- KALTOSTAT Wound Dressing
- Maxorb CMC/Alginate Dressing
- Sorbsan Topical Wound Dressing.

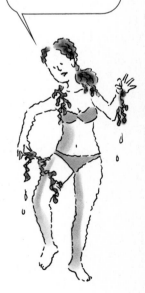

Alginate dressings are made from seaweed. Who knew this stuff was so useful?!

When they're used

Use alginate dressings on wounds with moderate to heavy drainage and wounds with tunneling.

What's the advantage?

Alginate dressings are beneficial because they:
- hold up to 20 times their own weight in fluid
- may be cut to fit wound dimensions
- may be layered for more absorption
- come in ropes for deep wound packing.

What to consider

Irrigation may be needed to remove an alginate dressing from the wound. In addition, alginate dressings:
- require secondary dressings
- can't be used on dry eschar or wounds with light drainage
- may dehydrate the wound bed of a dryer wound.

Antimicrobial dressings

Antimicrobial dressings protect against bacteria and provide a moist environment for wound healing—an improvement on topical antibiotic therapy. Active ingredients, such as silver, iodine, and polyhexethylene, provide the antimicrobial effects. These dressings come in many forms, including transparent dressings, gauze, island dressings, foams, and absorptive fillers.

Examples of antimicrobial dressings include:
- Acticoat
- AcryDerm Silver
- Iodosorb Gel
- SilverSorb.

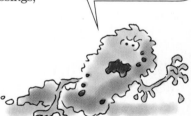

Drats! When a patient has an antimicrobial dressing in place, I don't stand a chance!

When they're used

Use antimicrobial dressings as primary or secondary dressings on wounds that are infected, draining, or nonhealing. You can also use them to manage minimal to heavy drainage.

What's the advantage?

Antimicrobial dressings:
- control bacteria
- help control odor
- work against a variety of microorganisms
- can often remain in place for 7 days.

What to consider

Antimicrobial dressings still require the patient to have systemic antibiotic therapy. In addition, antimicrobial dressings may:
• produce a hypersensitivity reaction in patients sensitive to such product ingredients as silver or iodine
• sting when applied
• contribute to the development of resistant organisms (not yet known)
• emit their own chemical odors.

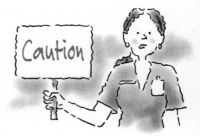

Biological dressings may help your patient's wound heal more quickly but beware of allergic reactions.

Biological dressings

Biological dressings are temporary dressings that function like skin grafts. They may be made from amnionic or chorionic membranes, woven from manmade fibers, or harvested from animals (usually pigs) or cadavers. Eventually, the body will reject a biological dressing. If rejection occurs before the underlying wound heals, the dressing must be replaced with a skin graft.

Examples of biological dressings include:
• Hyalofill Biopolymeric Wound Dressing
• Inerpan
• Oasis.

When they're used

Use biological dressings as temporary dressings for ulcers of varying thickness (depending on the product), skin grafting donor sites, and burns.

What's the advantage?

The biggest advantage of biological dressings is that they can shorten healing times. They also:
• prevent infection and fluid loss
• ease patient discomfort.

What to consider

Biological dressings:
• are relatively expensive
• may cause allergic reactions
• may require secondary dressings.

Collagen dressings

Collagen dressings, which are made from bovine or avian collagen, accelerate wound healing by encouraging the organization of new collagen fibers and granulation tissue. They're available in gel, granule, and sheet forms. Some also contain alginate.

Examples of collagen dressings include:
- FIBRACOL PLUS Collagen Wound Dressing with Alginate
- Kollagen-Medifil Pads.

When they're used

Use collagen dressings on chronic, nonhealing, granulated wound beds and wounds with tunneling.

What's the advantage?

Collagen dressings:
- are effective on chronic, clean wounds
- can be used on wounds with minimal to heavy drainage (depending on the product selected)
- are easy to apply.

What to consider

Collagen dressings aren't appropriate for third-degree burns or wounds with dry beds. In addition, they may:
- cause an allergic reaction if the patient is sensitive to collagen, bovine, or avian products
- require secondary dressings.

> *Collagen dressings are made from bovine or avian collagen. Remember that these dressings can cause an allergic reaction in patients sensitive to bovine or avian products.*

Composite dressings

Composite dressings are hybrid dressings that combine two or more types of dressings into one. For example, a three-layer composite dressing can include a bacterial barrier; an absorbent foam, hydrocolloid, or hydrogel layer; an adherent or a nonadherent layer; and an adhesive border.

Examples of composite dressings include:
- Alldress
- CompDress Island Dressing
- COVADERM Plus
- MPM Multi-Layered Dressing
- TELFA PLUS Island Dressing.

When they're used

Use composite dressing as primary or secondary dressings on wounds with minimal to heavy drainage. They can also be used to protect peripheral and central I.V. lines.

What's the advantage?

Composite dressings are:
• all-in-one dressings that come in various combinations to suit each patient's wound care needs
• available in multiple sizes and shapes.

What to consider

Composite dressings can't be used on third-degree burns. In addition, they:
• may not provide a moist wound environment (depending on the product selected) and may dry the wound bed
• can't be cut to fit without losing some of the dressing's integrity.

Contact layer dressings

Contact layer dressings are single-layer dressings made of woven or perforated material suitable for direct contact with the wound's surface. The nonadherent contact layer prevents other dressings from sticking to the surface of the wound.

Examples of contact layer dressings include:
• Conformant 2 Wound Veil
• Mepitel
• Profore Wound Contact Layer
• Telfa Clear.

When they're used

Use contact layer dressings to let drainage flow to a secondary dressing while preventing that dressing from adhering to the wound.

What's the advantage?

Contact layer dressings:
• decrease the pain experienced during dressing changes
• can be used with topical medications, fillers, and gauze dressings
• can be cut to fit or overlap the wound edges.

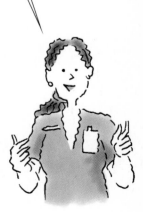

What a relief! Contact layer dressings decrease the pain experienced by the patient during dressing changes.

What to consider

Contact layer dressings require a secondary dressing and are contraindicated for use on third-degree burns, infected wounds, and wounds with tunneling.

Foam dressings

Foam dressings are nonadherent, somewhat absorbent spongelike polymer dressings that may include an adhesive border. They provide a moist healing environment and thermal insulation.

Examples of foam dressings include:
- Allevyn Cavity Wound Dressing
- CarraSmart Foam Dressing
- Hydrasorb Foam Wound Dressing
- Mepilex
- PolyTube Tube-Site Dressing
- Tielle Plus Hydropolymer Dressing.

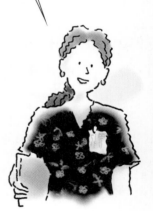

Use a foam dressing on a wound with minimal to moderate drainage when you need a nonadherent surface.

When they're used

Use foam dressings as primary or secondary dressings on wounds with minimal to moderate drainage (including around tubes) when you need a nonadherent surface.

What's the advantage?

Foam dressings may be used in combination with other products and those with an adhesive border don't require a secondary dressing. In addition, foam dressings:
- can be used on infected wounds if changed daily
- can manage heavier drainage because they wick moisture from the wound and allow evaporation (hydropolymer foam dressings)
- can be used around tubes (such as a tracheostomy) because they don't fray like gauze.

What to consider

Without an adhesive border, foam dressings may require a secondary dressing, tape, wrap, or net. In addition, they:
- have an adhesive border that may stick to the wound base
- can't manage large amounts of drainage
- may cause maceration if not changed regularly
- aren't recommended for nondraining wounds.

Hydrocolloid dressings

Hydrocolloid dressings are adhesive, moldable wafers made of a carbohydrate-based material. Most have a waterproof backing. They're impermeable to oxygen, water, and water vapor, and most provide some degree of absorption. These dressings turn to gel as they absorb moisture, help maintain a moist wound bed, and promote autolytic debridement.

Examples of hydrocolloid dressings include:
• BandAid Advanced Healing Bandages (available over-the-counter)
• DuoDERM CGF
• Restore Cx Wound Care Dressing
• 3M Tegasorb Hydrocolloid Dressing.

When they're used

Use hydrocolloid dressings on wounds with minimal to moderate drainage, including wounds with necrosis or slough. Hydrocolloid sheet dressings can also serve as secondary dressings.

What's the advantage?

Hydrocolloid dressings are beneficial because they:
• don't stick to a moist wound base
• maintain moisture by becoming gelatinous as they absorb drainage
• may require changing only two to three times each week
• can be easily removed from the wound base
• are available in contoured forms for use on specific sites
• are available in several varieties (sheets, powder, or gel) in thin and traditional thickness.

What to consider

Hydrocolloid dressings can't be used on burns or dry wounds. In addition, they:
• may have an odor when removed
• can cause skin stripping when removed
• can cause maceration or hypergranulation
• may need to be held in place to maximize adhesion.

Hydrogel dressings

Hydrogel dressings are water- or glycerin-based polymer dressings that don't adhere to wounds. They provide limited absorption (some are 96% water themselves) and are available as tubes of gel or in flexible sheets. Hydrogel dressings add moisture and promote autolytic debridement.

Examples of hydrogel dressings include:
- Aquasorb Hydrogel Wound Dressing
- Carrasyn Gel Wound Dressing with Acemannan Hydrogel
- CURASOL Gel Wound Dressing
- Hypergel
- Phyto Derma Wound Gel
- SAF-Gel Hydrating Dermal Wound Dressing
- TOE-AID Toe and Nail Dressing.

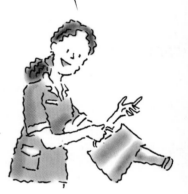

Using a hydrogel dressing is like watering a flower bed. The dressing provides moisture to the wound bed.

When they're used

Use hydrogel dressings on dry wounds, wounds with minimal drainage, or wounds with necrosis or slough.

What's the advantage?

Hydrogel dressings come in sheet and amorphous gel form. When applied, they may provide cooling that soothes and eases pain.

What to consider

Hydrogel dressings in gel form require a secondary dressing. Sterile gels are also expensive. In addition, they:
- can macerate surrounding skin
- may necessitate daily dressing changes
- vary in viscosity among brands and according to the product's base (water or glycerin).

Specialty absorptive dressings

Specialty absorptive dressings have multiple layers of a highly absorbent material, such as cotton or rayon, and may have adhesive borders. Various forms are available, including gels, pads, gauze, and pillows.

Examples of specialty absorptive dressings include:
- AQUACEL
- BreakAway Wound Dressing
- Sofsorb Wound Dressing
- TENDERSORB WET-PRUF Abdominal Pads.

When they're used

Use specialty absorptive dressings on infected or noninfected wounds with heavy drainage.

What's the advantage?

Specialty absorptive dressings:
- are highly absorbent (holding up to 33% more moisture than alginates)
- typically require less frequent changes
- are available in a variety of forms.

What to consider

Specialty absorptive dressings can't be used on burns or on wounds with little or no drainage.

Transparent film dressings

Transparent film dressings are clear, adherent, nonabsorptive, polyurethane dressings. They're semipermeable to oxygen and water vapor but not to water itself. Transparency allows visual inspection of the wound while the dressing is in place. Transparent film dressings maintain a moist wound environment and promote autolysis.

Examples of transparent film dressings include:
- BIOCLUSIVE Transparent Dressing
- BlisterFilm
- ClearSite Transparent Membrane
- OpSite FLEXIGRID
- 3M NexCare Waterproof Bandages (available over-the-counter)
- 3M Tegaderm Transparent Dressing.

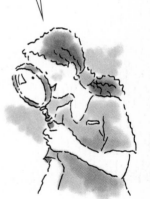

Transparent film dressings allow for visual inspection of the wound while the dressing is in place.

When they're used

Use transparent film dressings on partial-thickness wounds with minimal exudate and on wounds with eschar (dry, leathery, black necrotic tissue) to promote autolysis.

What's the advantage?

Transparent film dressings:
- may require less-frequent changes
- allow you to see the wound without removing the dressing
- are adherent but won't stick to the wound
- aren't bulky.

What to consider

Transparent film dressings don't absorb drainage, making them appropriate only for partial-thickness wounds or shallow, full-thickness wounds with minimal exudate. In addition, the adhesive border can strip skin around the wound when the dressing is removed.

Wound fillers

Wound fillers are specialized dressings used to fill deeper wounds. They're made of various materials and come in many forms, including pastes, granules, powders, beads, and gels. Wound fillers can add moisture to the wound bed or absorb drainage, depending on the product.

Examples of wound fillers include:
- AcryDerm STRANDS Absorbent Wound Filler
- Bard Absorption Dressing
- Catrix Wound Dressing
- Multidex Maltodextrin Wound Dressing Gel or Powder.

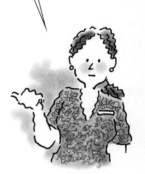

Remember, some wound fillers add moisture to the wound bed while others absorb drainage.

When they're used

Use wound fillers as primary dressings on infected or noninfected wounds with minimal to moderate drainage that require packing.

What's the advantage?

Wound fillers come in several forms with different absorption abilities.

What to consider

Wound fillers can't be used on third-degree burns, dry wounds, or wounds with tunnels and sinus tracts. Also, the wormlike appearance of some wound filler products can alarm a sensitive patient.

Adjunct wound care products

A wide variety of topical skin and wound care aids are available to complement the function of dressings. Products that directly impact the ability of a wound to heal include the Provant Wound Closure System, the Vacuum-Assisted Closure (VAC) device, the Warm-Up Therapy System, and debriding agents.

Provant Wound Closure System

The Provant Wound Closure System is a noninvasive treatment that stimulates healing by directly a treatment signal $2^3/4''$ to $3^1/8''$ (7 to 8 cm) into the tissues around the wound. This signal induces the proliferation of fibroblasts and epithelial cells as well as the secretion of multiple growth factors, resulting in faster healing.

Treatment doesn't require removal of existing dressings. Clinical studies indicate that the Provant system effectively promotes healing, even in cases of chronic, severe pressure ulcers.

When it's used

Use the Provant Wound Closure System on wounds in the inflammatory phase of healing.

What's the advantage?

The Provant Wound Closure System:
• requires no special training (patients may be able to perform therapy at home)
• requires only two 30-minute treatments per day (duration is pre-set in the device so it turns off automatically at the end of a session)
• may be used over existing dressings.

What to consider

The Provant system:
• can't be used for pregnant patients or those with cardiac pacemakers
• won't help heal bone or deep internal organs.

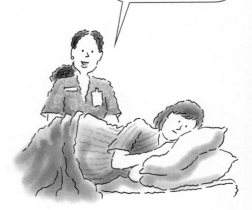

Remember, you can't use the Provant Wound Closure System on a pregnant patient.

Vacuum-Assisted Closure device

The VAC device uses negative air pressure to promote wound closure. VAC therapy, also called *negative pressure wound therapy*, can be used when a wound fails to heal in a timely manner. This system consists of a special open-cell polyurethane ether foam dressing cut to the size of the wound, a vacuum tube, and a vacuum pump. One end of the vacuum tube is placed over the foam dressing and the other connects to the vacuum pump. The dressing is sealed securely in place with adhesive tape that extends $1^1/4''$ to $2''$ (3 to 5 cm) over adjacent skin all around the dressing.

When turned on, the pump gently reduces air pressure beneath the dressing, drawing off exudate and reducing edema in surrounding tissues. This process reduces bacterial colonization, pro-

Understanding VAC therapy

Vacuum-assisted closure (VAC) therapy encourages healing by applying localized subatmospheric pressure at the site of the wound. This reduces edema and bacterial colonization and stimulates the formation of granulation tissue. This illustration shows the components of a VAC therapy device.

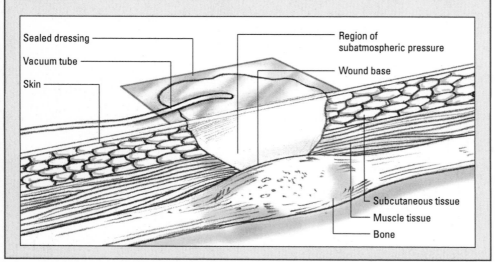

Sealed dressing

Vacuum tube

Skin

Region of subatmospheric pressure

Wound base

Subcutaneous tissue

Muscle tissue

Bone

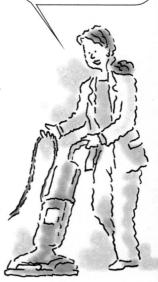

The VAC device aids healing by removing infectious drainage, promoting granulation tissue formation, and drawing wounds closed. If only it could help with the vacuuming!

motes granulation tissue development, increases the rate of cell mitosis, and spurs the migration of epithelial cells within the wound. Special training is required to operate this device. (See *Understanding VAC therapy.*)

Mini-me

An alternative is the MiniVAC device, a smaller, portable version that runs on rechargeable batteries and has a 50-ml drainage capacity.

Two additional VAC devices have recently been introduced:
• The VAC Freedom device is a portable, lightweight device with a 300-ml drainage capacity.
• The VAC-ATS, which is ideal for heavily draining wounds for patients in acute care settings, has touch-screen operations and a 500- to 1,000-ml drainage capacity.

When it's used

VAC therapy is useful in managing slow-healing acute, subacute, or chronic exudative wounds with cavities. It's ideal for pressure ulcers or surgical wounds with depths greater than 1 cm.

What's the advantage?

The VAC device:
• cleans deeply and can manage moderate to large amounts of drainage (VAC drainage capacity is 300 ml; MiniVAC, 50 ml; VAC Freedom, 300 ml; VAC-ATS, 500 to 1,000 ml.)
• can manage multiple wounds when dressings are cut to bridge two or more wounds (or when a Y-connector connects two wounds to one unit)
• has rechargeable batteries and is small enough to fit in a pouch that can be worn at the waist or over the shoulder (MiniVAC and VAC Freedom).

What to consider

VAC therapy is contraindicated for use with untreated osteo-myelitis, malignancies, and wounds with necrotic tissue or fistulas. In addition:
• the VAC vacuum tube is 5′ to 6′ (1.5 to 1.8 m) long, which requires that the patient remain in one place or carry the unit along
• the VAC and VAC-ATS devices require electricity; the MiniVAC and VAC Freedom batteries must be recharged frequently
• incorrect use of the VAC device, such as improperly setting the pressure, can result in bruising at the wound base.

Warm-Up Therapy System

The Warm-Up Therapy System, also called *noncontact normothermic wound therapy*, is a temporary therapy that increases the temperature of the wound bed, thereby promoting increased blood flow in the area of the wound. The dressing in this system contains a special electronic warming card. Once in place, the card heats to 100.4° F (38° C), bathing the wound in radiant heat. The closely sealed wound covering promotes a moist environment in the wound bed. This system is designed to remain in place for 72 hours.

The Warm-Up Therapy System increases the temperature of the wound bed, which increases blood flow in the wound area.

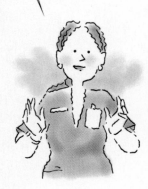

When it's used

As ordered, use the Warm-Up Therapy System on acute or chronic, full- or partial-thickness wounds, regardless of etiology, that have failed to heal with traditional therapies, including wounds with compromised blood flow, such as arterial or diabetic foot ulcers.

What's the advantage?

The Warm-Up Therapy System can absorb a small to moderate amount of drainage in the wound covering. In addition, it doesn't disturb the wound when removed and can be used on infected wounds.

What to consider

The Warm-Up Therapy System is contraindicated for use on third-degree burns. In addition, it requires specific dressings and thorough patient teaching related to dressing changes and heat management.

Debriding agents

When applied directly to necrotic or devitalized tissue, debriding agents (chemical or enzyme preparations) remove dead tissue in a wound. If the wound contains eschar, the eschar is crosshatched before application so the agent can penetrate the tissue.

Examples of debriding agents include:
- ACCUZYME
- Collagenase Santyl Ointment
- PANAFIL.

When they're used

Use debriding agents to debride wounds with moderate to large amounts of necrotic tissue, especially in cases where surgical debridement isn't an option.

What's the advantage?

Debriding agents may contain chlorophyll, which helps control odor; however, drainage may turn green and be wrongly interpreted as infection. In addition, they debride effectively even when used in small amounts.

What to consider

Debriding agents are expensive. In addition, they may:
- contain known allergens
- require secondary dressings
- cause irritation if they come in contact with surrounding skin
- cause a burning sensation in the wound during application that can last for several hours.

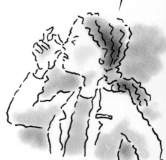

The chlorophyll found in some debriding agents helps to control wound odor.

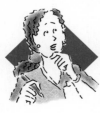

Quick quiz

1. What type of dressing is most appropriate for a patient with a dry wound?
    A.   Specialty absorptive
    B.   Amorphous hydrogel
    C.   Alginate
    D.   Foam

Answer: B. A dry wound needs added moisture to promote wound healing, so an amorphous hydrogel dressing should be used.

2. Which dressing type is most absorbent?
    A.   Hydrocolloid
    B.   Foam
    C.   Composite
    D.   Alginate

Answer: D. Although all of these products have some absorptive capacity, alginate dressings are the most absorbent.

3. What's the advantage of a debriding agent containing chlorophyll?
    A.   It can manage heavy exudate.
    B.   It controls bleeding.
    C.   It controls odor.
    D.   It speeds wound closure.

Answer: C. Chlorophyll helps reduce unpleasant odors.

4. You smell an unpleasant odor as you remove your patient's dressing. Which type of dressing may cause this finding?
    A.   Alginate
    B.   Hydrocolloid
    C.   Composite
    D.   Foam

Answer: B. Hydrocolloid dressings absorb drainage and turn to gel. This gel can have an unpleasant odor when exposed during dressing changes.

5.   Which wound care product uses negative air pressure to deep clean a wound?
- A.   VAC device
- B.   Warm-Up Therapy System
- C.   Debriding agent
- D.   Hydrocolloid dressing

Answer: A. The VAC device generates negative pressure that draws off exudate, bacteria, and excessive moisture.

Scoring

☆☆☆   If you answered all five questions correctly, shout it out! Your knowledge of wound care products is second to none.

☆☆   If you answered four questions correctly, we'd like to shake your hand! You've obviously absorbed all the material on wound care products.

☆   If you answered fewer than four questions correctly, that's okay! We'll count this one as warm-up therapy.

10

Therapeutic modalities

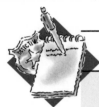

Just the facts

In this chapter, you'll learn:

♦ therapeutic modalities for wound healing

♦ physiologic effects of therapeutic modalities

♦ indications, contraindications, and application methods for therapeutic modalities.

A look at therapeutic modalities

Therapeutic modalities have commonly been described as adjunctive modalities — treatments that are used in addition to traditional therapies. However, this definition is slightly outdated today because therapeutic modalities are now part of standard care and are central to the wound healing process. (See *How therapeutic modalities promote healing*, page 218.)

Tradition!

Some therapeutic modalities, such as hydrotherapy and therapeutic light, have been used since the early 1900s. Many traditional modalities are still widely used today and new therapeutic modalities are always being developed.

New kids on the block

In many cases, new therapeutic modalities are based on traditional modalities. Some of the developing therapeutic modalities involve using near-infrared photo energy, inducing cell proliferation, and delivering ultrasound in a mist.

Selecting a therapeutic modality

To select the best therapeutic modalities for the patient, focus on his specific wound care needs. For example, if the wound needs

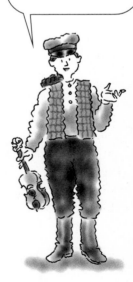

Traditional therapeutic modalities, such as hydrotherapy, have been in use since the 1900s. New treatments, often based on the traditional, continue to emerge.

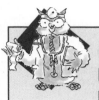

Get wise to wounds

How therapeutic modalities promote healing

Therapeutic modalities promote wound healing by:
• physically or mechanically debriding particulate and bacterial necrosis
• killing microorganisms or controlling bioburden (microorganism number)
• reducing or controlling edema and wound fluids
• increasing blood flow and tissue oxygenation
• enhancing immune or connective tissue cell function
• providing scaffolding for tissue growth.

debridement to remove necrosis and reduce microorganism counts, consider using:
• pulsatile lavage
• whirlpool
• electrical stimulation
• laser therapy
• ultraviolet (UV) treatment (using UVC radiation).

Lighten the load

For edema and lymphedema control and to reduce pathologic intercellular fluid loads, consider:
• electrical stimulation
• compression pumps or stockings.

Simply stimulating!

To stimulate tissue formation by increasing blood vessel formation (angiogenesis); to enhance blood flow and the delivery of oxygen, nutrients, and immune cells; to improve immune cell and wound bed cell function; and to stimulate wound matrix formation and collagen fiber alignment, the practitioner may order:
• growth factors
• living skin equivalents
• pulsatile lavage
• UV treatment (using UVA and UVB radiation)
• ultrasound
• electrical stimulation

Think about your patient's wound care needs. That's the key to selecting the best therapeutic modalities for each patient.

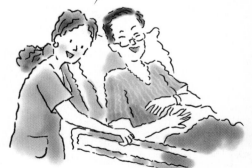

- laser therapy
- cell proliferation
- whirlpool.

Common therapeutic modalities

Therapeutic modalities widely embraced by today's wound care practitioners include:
- biotherapy (growth factors, living skin equivalents)
- hydrotherapy (pulsatile lavage, whirlpool)
- therapeutic light (UV treatment, laser therapy)
- ultrasound
- electrical stimulation
- hyperbaric oxygen.

Biotherapy

The biotherapy methods most commonly used in wound treatment include growth factors and living skin equivalents.

Growth factors

Growth factors are an important form of biotherapy because of the important role they play in the healing process (stimulating cell proliferation).

Getting the factors straight

Wound healing is a complex process that the body undertakes to replace or repair injured tissue. If various growth factors aren't synthesized, secreted, and removed from tissues with correct timing, the wound healing process can stall. This leaves the wound bed in a chronic state of confusion, unable to heal.

The master factor

In the past decade, growth factors have been studied to determine exactly how they function in healing and how they may be used in the treatment of chronic wounds. (See *Understanding growth factors*, page 220.) Particular focus has been placed on platelet-derived growth factor (PDGF), which some experts call the *master factor*. Although the specific growth factor or other mechanism that initiates wound healing isn't known, PDGF is known to play a central role by attracting fibroblasts (components of granulation tissue) and inducing them to divide. This is central to wound healing because fibroblasts are responsible for collagen formation.

> Growth factors stimulate cell proliferation, making them an important component of the healing process.

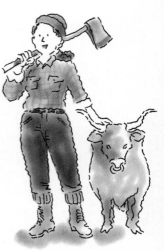

Understanding growth factors

This chart describes key growth factors that play an important role in wound healing.

Type	Description
TGF-ß (transforming growth factor beta)	Controls movement of cells to sites of inflammation and stimulates extracellular matrix formation
bFGF (basic fibroblast growth factor)	Stimulates angiogenesis (the development of blood vessels)
VEGF (vascular endothelial growth factor)	Stimulates angiogenesis
IGF (insulin–like growth factor)	Increases collagen synthesis
EGF (epidermal growth factor)	Stimulates epidermal regeneration

Trials and tribulations

The key growth factors PDGF, TGF-β, bFGF, and EGF have been through or are currently undergoing testing in clinical trials. At this time, the only synthetic growth factor approved for use in wound care is becaplermin (Regranex Gel 0.01%), which has a biological activity similar to that of endogenous PDGF. Regranex increases wound closure by 43%.

Dime-size dynamo

Regranex is recommended for use on lower-extremity diabetic neuropathic ulcers that have adequate blood flow and involve tissues at and below the subcutaneous level. It can be applied to wounds using a sterile applicator, such as a swab, a tongue blade, or saline-moistened gauze. A dime-size thickness of Regranex is all that's needed. The wound can then be dressed with a saline-moistened gauze. Keep in mind that Regranex is contraindicated in necrotic and infected wounds and in patients with poor blood supply to the legs.

Living skin equivalents

Another type of biotherapy available for chronic wound management involves the use of living skin equivalents, also called *tissue-engineered skin substitutes.*

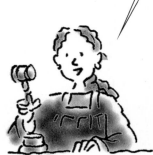

On trial today are the growth factors PDGF, TGF-β, bFGF, and EGF. Only becaplermin — a substance similar to PDGF — has been approved for use in wound care.

It's alive!

Living skin equivalents are living constructs derived from biological substances, such as bovine collagen and human neonatal foreskin. All living skin equivalents should be used on wounds with adequate blood flow that are free from infection and necrosis. Living skin equivalent is applied to a clean wound bed and several applications may be needed. This sterile procedure requires special training.

Two living skin equivalents approved by the Food and Drug Administration (FDA) in the United States are Dermagraft and graftskin (Apligraf). Be aware that these products are expensive, require special storage, and some have a short half-life. (See *Comparing living skin equivalents*.)

> Living skin equivalents are often made from bovine collagen.

Dermagraft

Dermagraft is a dermal substitute and, as such, is a single layer composed of human neonatal fibroblasts seeded on a polyglactin mesh (dissolvable suture material). The fibroblasts secrete and fill in this mesh with extracellular matrix. It's used to treat patients with partial-thickness burns and diabetic foot ulcers.

Dermagraft is contraindicated for use on clinically infected wounds and wounds with sinus tracks and in individuals with known allergies to bovine products.

Apligraf

Apligraf is a bilayered skin substitute consisting of an epidermal layer and a dermal layer. The dermal layer is composed of type 1 collagen and human neonatal fibroblasts; the epidermal layer is

Comparing living skin equivalents

Here's how two living skin equivalents measure up to each other.

Product	What it replaces	What it's made from	What it's used for
Dermagraft	Dermis	• Human fibroblasts on a polyglactin mesh	• Burns • Diabetic foot ulcers
Apligraf	Epidermis and dermis	• Type 1 collagen • Human fibroblasts • Human keratinocytes	• Venous ulcers • Diabetic foot ulcers

formed from human keratinocytes (the epidermal cells that synthesize keratin). Apligraf is approved for use in both venous and diabetic foot ulcers.

When applied to venous ulcers, Apligraf is used along with standard compression therapy. For a patient with a diabetic foot ulcer, appropriate off-loading devices are also used.

Contraindications for Apligraf include use on wounds that are infected and use in individuals with known allergies to bovine collagen or other components in the medium in which Apligraf is shipped.

Hydrotherapy

One of the oldest therapeutic modalities, hydrotherapy is used in wound care by members of many disciplines (such as physical therapy). It can take various forms, including:
- pulsatile lavage with concurrent suction
- whirlpool therapy
- jet irrigation
- irrigation with a bulb syringe or a syringe with an attached angiocatheter.

As with most treatments, the type of therapy used depends on the patient's wound type.

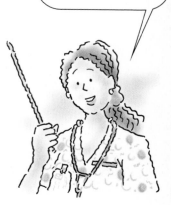

Pulsatile lavage has several advantages, including improved comfort for the patient and effectiveness in reaching deep tunneling in wounds.

Pulsatile lavage

Today, most hydrotherapy treatments are delivered by pulsatile lavage. Pulsatile lavage cleans and debrides wounds by combining pulse irrigation with suction.

Advantages of using pulsatile lavage include:
- improved comfort for the patient
- mobility of the apparatus (can be performed in a hospital, clinic, or home setting)
- effectiveness in reaching deep, tunneling wounds
- minimized chance of cross-contamination.

Additionally, at least one preliminary study suggests that pulsatile lavage promotes the formation of granulation tissue.

Versatility is a virtue

Pulsatile lavage can be used with almost any wound type: acute or chronic, large or small, infected or noninfected, and clean or necrotic.

Indications for pulsatile lavage include:
- clean wounds—to increase granulation tissue formation
- slow-healing wounds—to increase granulation tissue formation

- infected or heavily contaminated wounds — to decrease bioburden levels
- wound bed preparation — for grafting with either skin grafts or living skin equivalents
- removal of necrotic tissue or other particulate.

Puttin' on the spritz

Sterile normal saline solution at room temperature is typically used for pulsatile lavage. It's applied by spray gun using a plastic, disposable fan tip. A tunneling tip is used for deep wounds with tunnels or extensive undermining.

The solution is delivered under pressure to the wound bed and concurrently aspirated by negative pressure through a separate plastic tube in the spray gun. The therapist can control both the delivery or impact pressure of the sterile normal saline solution and the suction pressure for aspiration of the contaminated fluid. (See *Pressures for pulsatile lavage.*)

Pressures for pulsatile lavage

The amount of pressure used for pulsatile lavage depends on the patient's wound type:

- High impact and suction pressures are used for dirty, necrotic wounds.
- Intermediate pressures are used for infected wounds.
- Low pressures are used for clean, granulating wounds.

Specific impact, or delivery pressures, and suction pressures are listed below.

Wound type	Impact pressure*	Suction pressure
Clean or granulating	4 to 8 psi	60 to 80 mm Hg
Infected	8 to 10 psi	80 to 100 mm Hg
Necrotic	10 to 12 psi	100 to 120 mm Hg

*Note: Impact pressures of less than 15 psi are recommended for wound management. Nonphysician providers shouldn't exceed an impact pressure of 15 psi without on-site supervision by a physician or a specific order for this pressure level.

Pulsatile precautions

Currently, no recognized contraindications for pulsatile lavage exist; however, you should consider premedicating the patient with analgesia for comfort during the procedure. Suggested precautions include:
- using lower impact and suction pressures on fragile tissue
- avoiding direct pressure over exposed nerves and blood vessels
- avoiding high-impact pressure over malignant tissue
- avoiding high-impact and suction pressures and static delivery in areas where excess suction may draw tissue into the tip as well as over grafts and exposed organs and body cavities.

Whirlpool therapy

In whirlpool therapy, part of the patient's body is immersed in a tank of water that has been heated to a prescribed temperature and circulated by an agitator. This therapy softens tissue, removes debris and drainage, and improves blood flow to the area, enhancing the delivery of oxygen and nutrients. Treatment times range from 10 to 20 minutes. A whirlpool tank may also be used for exercise therapy for patients with open wounds or when a therapeutic pool isn't available.

Size matters

Whirlpool tanks are available in several sizes: small tanks for hands and extremities, medium-sized tanks for lower body treatments, and large tanks for upper and lower body treatments.

When to whirl

Whirlpool therapy is useful for large surface area treatments, especially when these areas are covered with tough necrotic tissue. Whirlpool treatments are also useful with painful ulcers when the patient can't tolerate the pressure of a pulsatile lavage head or when allergies to local anesthetics prevent the use of pulsatile lavage.

Indications for whirlpool treatment include:
- large surface area wounds
- wounds with tough, black eschar
- wounds with particulate (such as "road rash")
- painful wounds.

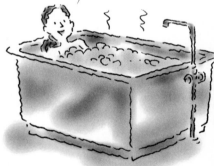

Whirlpool tanks come in several sizes, depending on the area of the body that needs treatment.

Temperature temperance

The temperature ranges used in whirlpool therapy are:
- tepid or nonthermal—80° to 92° F (26.7° to 33.3° C)
- neutral (local skin temperature)—92° to 96° F (35.6° C)
- warm or thermal—96° to 104° F (40° C).

The appropriate water temperature depends on the patient's wound type:
- For arterial wounds, a neutral temperature is recommended, along with shorter treatment times (2 to 5 minutes) so as not to increase tissue metabolism in an ischemic limb.
- For venous ulcers, tepid whirlpool temperature and short treatment times (2 to 5 minutes) are recommended because the edema associated with venous ulcers may increase with warm or hot whirlpool for extended treatments due to both heat exposure and the dependent position of the lower extremities.
- For pressure ulcers and other types of wounds, neutral to warm temperatures are recommended. Warm temperatures may inactivate the harmful enzymes in chronic wound beds.

Everyone else, out of the pool!

Contraindications to whirlpool include:
- wound infections
- edema
- deep vein thrombosis or acute phlebitis
- cardiovascular, pulmonary, or renal failure
- unresponsiveness or dementia
- bowel or bladder incontinence
- wounds with dry gangrene.

Therapeutic light

In therapeutic light modalities, light or its energy is used to aid in wound healing. The modalities include UV treatment and laser therapy.

UV treatment

Although not a form of light, UV energy or radiation is commonly categorized as therapeutic light. UV energy lies between X-rays and visible light on the electromagnetic spectrum. It has been used for more than 100 years for the treatment of slow healing and infected wounds. Heliotherapy, or sun therapy, has most likely been used since the dawn of humankind for skin problems and other health care needs.

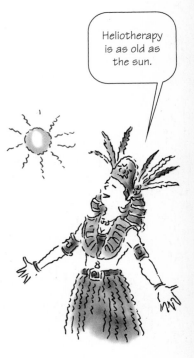

Heliotherapy is as old as the sun.

Strike up the bands

UV radiation is typically divided into three bands: UVA, UVB, and UVC. Here are some benefits of treatment with UVA and UVB radiation:
• Chronic pressure ulcers treated with UVA and UVB energy have exhibited increased wound healing in clinical studies.
• UVA and UVB energy enhance white blood cell (WBC) accumulation and lysosomal activity, possibly offering an explanation for UV-mediated debridement.
• UV radiation stimulates the production of interleukin-1 alpha, a cytokine that plays a role in epithelialization.

The utility of UVC has been demonstrated in various wound types. It's primarily used for treatment in patients with infected wounds. An added benefit of UVC is that it kills a broad spectrum of microorganisms with low exposure times and isn't likely to generate resistant microorganisms. Recent research has shown that UVC can kill antibiotic-resistant strains of bacteria, such as methicillin-resistant *Staphylococcus aureus*. UVC is easily administered with minimal intervention time and its also inexpensive. (See *Application of UVC radiation*.)

UV utility

Indications for UV treatment include:
• chronic, slow healing wounds
• infected or heavily contaminated wounds
• necrotic wounds.

Contraindications for UV treatment include certain chronic disease states, such as:
• diabetes
• pulmonary tuberculosis
• hyperthyroidism
• systemic lupus erythematosus
• cardiac disease
• renal disease
• hepatic disease
• acute eczema
• herpes simplex.

Laser therapy

The word "laser" is actually an acronym for light amplification by stimulated emission of radiation. Lasers can be divided into two groups:
• Cold lasers include the helium neon, or red laser, and the gallium-arsenide laser.

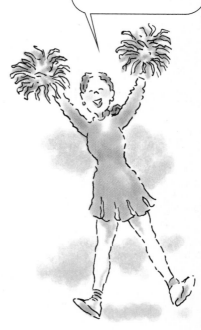

Gimme an L!
Gimme an A!
Gimme an S-E-R!
What does it spell?
LASER! What does it stand for? Light amplification by stimulated emission of radiation!

Application of UVC radiation

Primarily used to treat patients with infected wounds, ultraviolet C (UVC) radiation kills a broad spectrum of microorganisms with low exposure times. Here's how it's used.

Cover-up
First, the skin around the wound is protected with a thick application of UV-impenetrable ointment, such as zinc oxide or petroleum. Other skin areas are covered with clean sheets. The eyes of the patient and the person administering the therapy must be covered with UV protective glasses.

Turn-on
The UVC lamp is then placed 1″ (2.5 cm) from the surface and then turned on for 30 to 60 seconds. This is done once daily for about 1 week or until the infection has cleared. Fungal infections may require a slightly longer treatment time (90 seconds).

Space-out
Tissue spacers, as shown below, may be added to maintain the appropriate distance of the lamp from the wound.

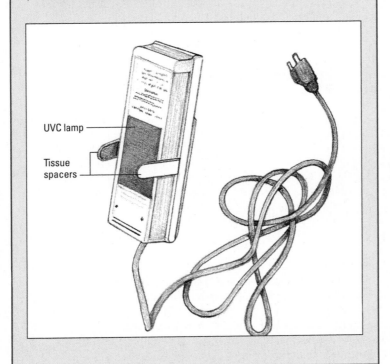

UVC lamp

Tissue spacers

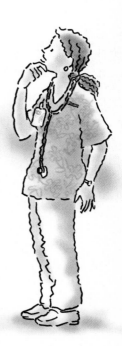

- Hot lasers encompass the carbon dioxide laser and other lasers used for surgical dissection.

In wound healing, cold lasers promote wound closure and nerve regeneration. The treatment consists of either placing the laser probe directly over selected treatment points for a specific time, according to the dosage required, or using a gridlike pattern and continuously moving the probe over this grid for a specific treatment time.

Laser tag

Indications for cold laser therapy include:
- slow healing wounds
- nerve regeneration
- pain relief.

Contraindications for cold laser therapy include treatments over:
- the eye
- a hemorrhage
- a malignancy
- a pregnant woman's uterus
- photosensitive skin.

Ultrasound

Ultrasound (mechanical pressure waves) is used in treatments for patients with both open and closed wounds because of its non-thermal and thermal effects. Ultrasound appears to have optimal effects when used during the inflammatory phase of wound healing. It speeds the wound's progress through the healing phases.

Cavitation sensation

Nonthermal effects of ultrasound include acoustic cavitation and microstreaming.
- In acoustic cavitation, gaseous bubbles are made to expand and contract rhythmically in the tissues being treated. These bubbles are thought to stimulate biological phenomena such as the activation of ionic channels in cellular membranes.
- Microstreaming is another nonthermal effect that results from cavitation. Cavitation causes fluids close to the bubbles to stream by, thus stimulating the cells in close proximity. In this way, ultrasound increases calcium conductance in fibroblasts, which is important because collagen secretion is a calcium-dependent process.

Ultrasound aids wound healing nonthermally through acoustic cavitation and microstreaming. It's all about the bubbles.

Gets the blood flowing

Ultrasound's thermal effects include increased blood flow to tissue, which results in increased tissue healing. Ultrasound also increases WBC migration and promotes a more orderly arrangement of collagen in both open and closed wounds.

This might be a job for ultrasound

Ultrasound is indicated to:
• increase wound healing
• enhance blood flow
• decrease pain
• decrease inflammation.
　　Contraindications for ultrasound include:
• malignant tissue
• acute infections
• deep vein thrombosis
• ischemic areas
• plastic implants or implanted electronic devices
• irradiated areas
• treatment over the gonads, spinal cord, eyes, or a pregnant woman's uterus.

Electrical stimulation

Electrical stimulation is used to enhance healing of recalcitrant wounds, especially chronic pressure ulcers. The types of electrical stimulation used in wound healing include high-voltage and low-voltage pulsed current. Electrical stimulation is delivered through a device that has conductive electrodes, which are applied to the skin.

Zap it!

Electrical stimulation can be used to:
• promote wound healing
• orient cells
• promote cellular migration
• enhance blood flow
• increase protein synthesis and wound bed formation
• destroy microorganisms
• increase angiogenesis
• increase tissue oxygenation
• reduce wound bioburden or microbial content
• reduce pain (wound and diabetic neuropathic pain).

Lack of stimulation

Contraindications for electrical stimulation include:
- malignant tissue
- untreated osteomyelitis
- treatment over pericardial area or areas related to control of cardiac and respiratory function
- treatment over some implanted electronic devices.

Hyperbaric oxygen

Hyperbaric oxygen (HBO) is the delivery of 100% oxygen through a sealed chamber. Two forms of HBO are used for wound healing. One form involves a total body chamber, such as that used for decompression therapy for divers, and the other involves a smaller chamber used just for the limbs. (The effectiveness of topical HBO through small-limb chambers hasn't been proven through research.)

In demand

HBO delivered by a whole body chamber increases the amount of dissolved oxygen in the blood that's available for wound healing. This increased availability of readily available oxygen in the blood can be used by cells, such as neutrophils, that employ oxygen-dependent processes. (The processes by which neutrophils destroy microorganisms are oxygen-based, as is cellular metabolism in general). In addition, the increased availability of oxygen for tissues apparently relieves relative hypoxia in wounded tissues.

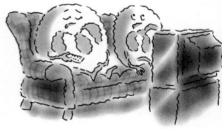

HBO a go!

Evidence supporting systemic or whole body HBO treatment for patients with chronic wounds is evolving. Patients with venous ulcers that don't improve with traditional therapies may benefit when compression therapy is paired with systemic HBO treatment. Another possible use for HBO is in treating patients with diabetic foot ulcers. HBO increases nitric oxide production in the wound. Nitric oxide is a unique free radical that's important in vasodilation and neurotransmission, which play major roles in diabetic wound healing.

However, keep in mind that HBO is contraindicated for patients taking antineoplastic agents or who are experiencing pneumothorax.

New therapeutic modalities

Several new therapeutic modalities for wound care have evolved in the past decade. Recent developments that are new to the market or haven't yet reached the market are:

- monochromatic near-infrared photo energy (MIRE)
- cell proliferation induction (CPI)
- mist ultrasound transport therapy (MUST).

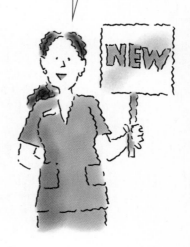

New therapeutic modalities include MIRE, CPI, and MUST.

You'll adMIRE this!

Treatment with MIRE is approved by the FDA for increasing circulation and reducing pain. The nitric oxide that's released into the bloodstream when MIRE is applied to the skin increases blood flow, delivering nutrients to the area and promoting healing. Neural function (sensation) may also improve due to increased blood flow to impaired nerves.

Sending the right signal

CPI technology involves the use of a low-level, confined, radiofrequency signal to stimulate wound healing. The signal is delivered at or near the cycle time for calcium channels, thus inducing the release of growth factors by a calcium-dependent mechanism. CPI has been shown to increase the proliferation of fibroblasts and epithelial cells and has been found to stimulate wound closure in pressure wounds.

This mist is a MUST

In MUST, ultrasound energy is transferred directly to the wound through a sterile saline mist. MUST enhances wound healing and decreases bacterial and necrotic debris in tissue by:

- enhancing fibroblast migration rates (shown in the laboratory)
- increasing collagen levels (shown in an animal wound model)
- decreasing bacterial numbers (shown in the laboratory and a patient case study)
- enhancing blood flow.

The minds, they are a-changin'

These new technologies represent a recent trend in thinking about chronic wound management — that is, that the cells normally involved in wound healing should be stimulated as part of wound care. By doing this, cells are encouraged to do what they do best: orchestrate the complex cascade of events that lead to wound healing.

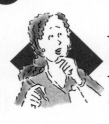

Quick quiz

1. Which growth factor is marketed as Regranex?
A. TGF-β
B. PDGF
C. IGF
D. VEGF

Answer: B. Becaplermin (Regranex Gel 0.01%) is the only genetically engineered growth factor substance approved by the FDA for use in wound care. It has a biological activity similar to that of PDGF produced by the body.

2. Which type of hydrotherapy is used most commonly for wound care?
A. Pulsatile lavage
B. Whirlpool
C. Jet irrigation devices
D. Bulb syringe

Answer: A. Today, most hydrotherapy treatments are delivered by pulsatile lavage because of improved comfort for the patient; the mobility of the apparatus; its ability to reach deep, tunneling wounds; the minimal chance for cross-contamination; and the decreased physical and departmental resources required for treatment.

3. What whirlpool temperature should be used for the patient with a venous ulcer?
A. Cold
B. Tepid
C. Warm
D. Hot

Answer: B. Tepid whirlpool temperature (80° to 92° F [26.7° to 33.3° C]) is recommended for venous ulcers because the edema associated with venous ulcers may increase with warm or hot whirlpool temperature. Cold water isn't recommended.

4. What type of UV light is used for infected wounds?
A. UVA
B. UVB
C. UVC
D. UVD

Answer: C. UVC is primarily used for the treatment of infected wounds because it kills a broad range of microorganisms with short exposure times. Also, it isn't likely to generate resistant microorganisms.

5. What's the maximum recommended impact pressure for pulsatile lavage?
- A. 5 psi
- B. 10 psi
- C. 15 psi
- D. 20 psi

Answer: C. Unless there's a specific order for a higher impact pressure or a doctor is present to supervise, impact pressure shouldn't exceed 15 psi.

6. Which type of therapy increases the amount of dissolved oxygen in the blood?
- A. Ultrasound
- B. Electrical stimulation
- C. Laser
- D. HBO

Answer: D. By increasing the amount of dissolved oxygen in the blood, HBO therapy increases the availability of oxygen to wounded tissues, which improves healing.

7. Which condition is contraindicated for the use of electrical stimulation?
- A. Untreated osteomyelitis
- B. Chronic pressure ulcers
- C. Decreased tissue oxygenation
- D. Decreased blood flow

Answer: A. Electrical stimulation is contraindicated for a patient with untreated osteomyelitis.

8. Which type of growth factor increases collagen synthesis during wound healing?
- A. VEGF
- B. IGF
- C. EGF
- D. bFGF

Answer: B. IGF plays an important role in wound healing by increasing collagen synthesis.

Scoring

☆☆☆   If you answered all eight questions correctly, take a bow! You're sizzling hot when it comes to therapeutic modalities.

☆☆   If you answered five to seven questions correctly, don't give up! Time and a quick review will heal your wounded pride.

☆   If you answered fewer than five questions correctly, maybe you whirled through the information too quickly! Review the chapter and try again.

Legal and reimbursement issues

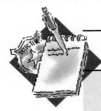

Just the facts

In this chapter, you'll learn:

◆ legal and reimbursement issues related to wound care

◆ established standards for health care practice, including Agency for Healthcare Research and Quality guidelines and state practice acts

◆ documentation strategies that can help you avoid litigation.

A look at legal and reimbursement issues

Wounds affect thousands of people each year. They contribute to morbidity and mortality, increase the cost of care and, sometimes, contribute to liability issues. To safeguard your practice, you need to know to what standards you're held in the event of a legal issue. By learning to properly evaluate wounds, you can dramatically improve your wound care patients' clinical and financial outcomes. At the same time, you'll avoid legal traps and denial of reimbursement.

What's a legal issue?

A legal issue is anything questionable in provided care that's related to some adverse occurrence or outcome.

Sticking to the issues

Here are some examples of legal issues:
• a possibly negligent action or omission by a health care provider
• deviation from an accepted standard of care
• inconsistencies in documentation.

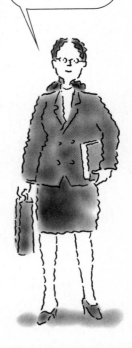

A legal issue is anything questionable in the care you provide that leads to an adverse outcome.

A common question that arises in issues of medical malpractice is, "Has the clinician met accepted standards of care?" For example, did a wound care specialist fail to implement preventive measures even though a patient was identified as being at risk for pressure ulcers?

Standards of care

Standard of care is a term used to specify what's reasonable under a certain set of circumstances. Standards are used to define certain aspects of a profession, such as:
• the focus of its pursuits
• the beneficiaries of its service
• the responsibilities of its practitioners.
    In health care, the prevailing professional standard of care is defined as the level of care, skill, and treatment deemed acceptable and appropriate by similar health care providers. A standard is a yardstick against which effective care can be measured.

Standard issue

The standards for wound care practice are derived from several sources:
• Agency for Healthcare Research and Quality (AHRQ) guidelines
• *Patient Care Partnership*
• facility- and unit-specific policies and procedures
• job descriptions
• American Nurses Association (ANA) *Standards of Clinical Nursing Practice*
• state nurse practice acts and guidelines.

Agency for Healthcare Research and Quality guidelines

Guidelines from the AHRQ — formerly the Agency for Health Care Policy and Research (AHCPR) — are a primary source of wound care standards for all health care practitioners. The AHRQ supports research and provides evidence-based information related to health care. (See *Spotlight on the AHRQ*.)

An ounce of prevention...

In the past decade, numerous campaigns have focused on establishing and publishing best-practice guidelines for pressure ulcer prevention and treatment. In the 1990s, the AHRQ (then the AHCPR) sponsored the *Clinical Practice Guidelines* for effective and appropriate care of specific patient populations. Two are specific to wound care:

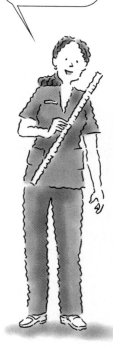

How do you measure up? A standard of care is the yardstick used to measure effectiveness of care.

Spotlight on the AHRQ

The Agency for Healthcare Research and Quality (AHRQ) is a federal agency that sponsors and conducts research on major areas of health care, including:
- quality improvement and patient safety
- outcomes and effectiveness of care
- clinical practice and technology assessment
- health care organization and delivery systems
- health care costs and sources of payment.

- *Prevention of Pressure Ulcers* (AHCPR *Clinical Practice Guideline* number 3) deals with tools to identify patients at risk for developing pressure ulcers and guidelines for basic preventive skin care and early treatment.
- *Treatment of Pressure Ulcers* (AHCPR *Clinical Practice Guideline* number 15) provides specific aspects of pressure ulcer care and corresponding evidence to support each recommendation.

Patient Care Partnership

The *Patient Care Partnership* (formerly known as the *Patient's Bill of Rights*) is another recognized basis for standards of care.

We, the people...

The American Hospital Association (AHA) first sanctioned the *Patient's Bill of Rights* in 1973 to establish the standards of treatment that each patient can expect. In 2002, the AHA replaced the *Patient's Bill of Rights* with the *Patient Care Partnership*. It includes the patient's right to:
- considerate and respectful care
- know, by name, the practitioner accountable for his care and to acquire from the practitioner thorough information related to his diagnosis, treatment, and prognosis
- receive enough information to give informed consent
- refuse treatment
- privacy relative to his medical care
- confidentiality
- solicit hospital services even if it means evaluation and referral to an accepting hospital
- acquire information such as the names of individuals involved in providing his care

- be informed if the hospital plans to engage in experimental treatment and the right to refuse to partake in such treatment
- expect follow-up care on discharge
- review and receive an explanation of his bill
- understand hospital rules and regulations related to patient conduct.

Facility- and unit-specific policies and procedures

The policies and procedures in your facility are also used to establish standards of care. Policies and procedures are commonly used in litigation claims. Too often, practitioners are informed of policies and procedures but don't take time to examine and understand them. Deviating from facility policies and procedures suggests failure to meet the facility's standards of care.

Job descriptions

Job descriptions play a role in determining standards of care as well. How does your employer define the health care team's roles and relationships? Depending on the practice setting—such as hospital, home, or extended care facility—your role may vary.

That's not in my job description!

To protect patients and staff members, firm practice guidelines are needed for all personnel to make sure that job descriptions are accurate. If health care employees practice outside their formal job descriptions, the facility's legal counsel or the insurance company could win a judgment against those employees to recover some of the losses incurred.

Standards of Clinical Nursing Practice

For professional nursing, the ANA's *Standards of Clinical Nursing Practice* outline the expectations of the comprehensive professional role within which all nurses must practice. Nursing practice standards ensure that the quality of nursing care, documentation, consistency, accountability, and professional credibility are upheld.

To each his own

The ANA first published the *Standards of Nursing Practice* in 1973. Since then, specialty nursing organizations have developed their own standards of practice in various areas of nursing, such as in emergency, perioperative, oncologic, and critical care nurs-

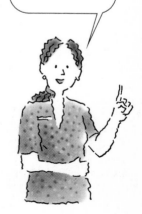

Nursing care specialists must live up to high standards established by specialty nursing organizations.

ing. Some of these standards were developed and published in collaboration with the ANA.

In 1991, the *Standards of Nursing Practice* was revised with participation from state nurses associations and specialty nursing organizations. The revised publication—*Standards of Clinical Nursing Practice*—is a comprehensive outline of expectations for all nurses. *Standards of Clinical Nursing Practice* is composed of authoritative statements describing a level of care or performance common to the nursing profession. It sets a standard by which the quality of nursing practice can be judged.

Expert standards

The Wound, Ostomy, and Continence Nurses Society (WOCN) is the professional organization for wound, ostomy, and continence (WOC) nurses (formerly known as *enterostomal nurses*). WOC nurses are experts in skin care and wound management. In 1987, the WOCN standards of care were developed for patients with dermal wounds (pressure sores and leg ulcers). Since then, the standards have been revised to reflect advances in technology and updated research findings.

State nurse practice acts and guidelines

Nurse practice acts and guidelines set by each state are also used to establish standards of care for nurses.

Act-ually, they're laws

State nurse practice acts are laws that define which treatments, actions, and functions can be performed or delegated in each state.

For example, conservative sharp debridement is a method of removing loose, nonviable tissue with sterile instruments. According to most state nurse practice acts, it may be performed by "trained health care professionals" such as registered nurses. The range of a nurse's legal responsibilities regarding conservative sharp debridement may vary from state to state. It's each nurse's professional responsibility to understand her scope of practice. If a nurse is licensed in more than one state, she needs to make sure that she's familiar with the specific guidelines of the state in which she's practicing.

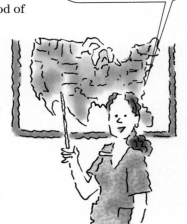

Location is relevant for nurses. A nurse must make sure she's familiar with the guidelines of the state in which she's practicing.

Litigation

Litigation is a lawsuit that's contested in court to enforce a right or pursue a resolution. Examples of legal liability specifically related to wound care usually involve claims of negligence, such as:

- failure to prevent
- failure to treat
- failure to heal.

Negligence, which is now recognized as a form of malpractice, is defined as failure to meet a standard of care — in other words, failure to do what another reasonably prudent health care provider would do in similar circumstances.

More and more

Practitioners are being sued individually for malpractice with increasing frequency. Malpractice is a health care professional's wrongful conduct, improper discharge of professional duties, or failure to meet standards of care that result in harm to another person. Most malpractice litigation comes as a result of claims that a health care provider failed to:

- provide physical protection
- monitor or assess
- promptly respond
- properly administer a medication.

Practitioners in critical care, emergency, trauma, and obstetrics and those who practice as specialists are most vulnerable.

ABCDs of medical malpractice

Four criteria must be verified to determine whether a medical malpractice claim is merited:

A duty must be established with the patient. What this means is that the practitioner accepts *accountability* for the care and treatment of the patient.

A *breach of duty* or *standard of care* by the practitioner must be determined to evaluate if there has been an act of negligence or breach of duty that resulted in harm to the patient.

Proximate cause or *causal connection* must be established between the breach of duty or standard of care and the damages or injuries to the patient. In other words, the patient must prove that damages were due directly to the practitioner's negligence and that the damages were foreseeable. In other words, were the damages a direct result of the negligence?

Damages or *injuries* to the patient must be presented as evidence as a result of the alleged negligence. These damages can be physical (disfigurement or pain and suffering), mental (mental anguish), or financial (past, present, or future medical expenses).

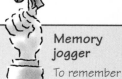

Memory jogger

To remember the four criteria that merit a medical malpractice claim, think **ABCD**:

Accountability rests with the practitioner.

Breach of duty leads to damages.

Causal connection is established between the breach and the damages.

Damages or injuries are presented as evidence of the breach of duty.

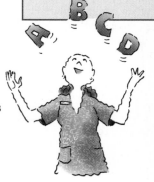

If the patient-plaintiff can establish these four components, malpractice litigation is merited.

> Practicing without your own malpractice insurance is risky. The insurance company that covers your employer may be more allegiant to the employer than to you.

Avoiding litigation

The key to reducing your risk of involvement in malpractice litigation is prevention. However, even if you provide optimum care to every patient, there's no guarantee that your actions will never be called into question in a litigation case. If that happens, you must be aware of how you're protected.

A common misconception

Many practitioners practice under the perception that they're protected by their facility's or employer's insurance policy. In most legal claims, your interests and the interests of your employer are comparable. However, the insurance company that provides your employer's coverage may be more allegiant to the employer than to you. In addition, the employer's insurance may not cover you if your performance fell outside your job description or if you didn't follow written policy and procedure.

Practicing without your own malpractice insurance is risky. Malpractice insurance doesn't keep you from getting sued, but it may lift most of the financial burden and fear of a lawsuit off your shoulders. Remember, it's expensive to prove your innocence.

The best defense

Excellent documentation is the key to minimizing your liability because it's direct evidence of your evaluation and care related to wounds. The medical record is your best protection and first line of defense. (See *Documentation do's and don'ts*, page 242.)

At your service

A patient's satisfaction with care also reduces liability. Typically, a malpractice claim represents the connection between patient injury and patient anger. Good communication with the patient and his family is essential to maintaining a good connection.

Health care is a service industry, so you need to incorporate good customer service into your daily practice, including:
• being respectful and courteous — People become angry when treated rudely.
• being attentive — Give the patients the time that they need.

Documentation do's and don'ts

To protect yourself against liability, document as accurately as possible by following these guidelines.

Do
• Chart factually, specifically, and concisely — Present your observations and interventions clearly and concisely.
• Chart thoroughly — Malpractice claims are commonly filed years later and the passage of time impairs your ability to remember details.
• Chart promptly — Making tardy or late entries may lead to inadvertent omissions.

Don't
• Chart personal observations, opinions, feelings, or beliefs — These aspects of care are irrelevant.

Make sure you dish up a healthy serving of respectful attention to every customer.

• being sympathetic and empathetic — Concern pays off in the long run.
• being considerate and honest — Patients recognize honesty, which makes them feel better about the care they receive.
• recognizing your limits — Ask for help or a second opinion if you have doubts.
• staying current — Continuing education is a professional responsibility.

Reimbursement

Understanding finances as they relate to wound care is essential when you're providing care to high-risk patients and those with alterations in skin integrity, such as an ulcer or a wound. Why? Because treating wounds can be costly.

Dollars and sense

With the ever-increasing costs of health care, it's time to recognize your role when it comes to reimbursement. Putting cost-effective wound care into clinical practice requires knowledge of payment systems and documentation strategies.

Payment systems

The language of health insurance is complicated; make sure you can recognize basic terms related to payment systems.

Examples of payment systems include:

- Medicare
- Medicaid
- managed care
- private pay.

Medicare

Medicare is a federal insurance program for people age 65 and older, specific disabled individuals, and people with diagnosed end-stage renal disease. It's administered by the Centers for Medicare and Medicaid Services (CMS).

Medicare A to B

Medicare is split into part A (hospital insurance) and part B (medical insurance):

- Part A coverage encompasses inpatient hospital care, inpatient skilled nursing facility care associated with inpatient hospitalization, home health care after inpatient hospitalization, and hospice care.
- Part B coverage includes services provided by doctors and other health care professionals, ambulance services, and durable medical supplies and equipment (such as wound care dressings and other supplies). (See *Guidelines for Medicare coverage of surgical dressings*.)

Who's picking up the check?

CMS contracts with insurance companies to process and pay claims for health care provided to Medicare beneficiaries. Payment for services and products varies according to practice settings, such as acute care hospitals, skilled nursing facilities, home health care agencies, outpatient facilities, and hospices.

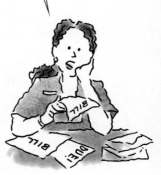

Make sure you understand the basics of payment systems, which include Medicare and Medicaid.

Guidelines for Medicare coverage of surgical dressings

Medicare covers surgical dressings for patients who:

- need them to treat a wound caused by surgery or surgical procedures
- need them after wound cleaning
- have severe bedsores or ulcers.

These patients must also meet certain requirements to be eligible for reimbursement. They must:

- have a prescription that's signed and dated by the prescriber
- be enrolled in Medicare and have a supplier number.

Recognizing reimbursement terms

Being aware of some of the terms associated with reimbursement for care, services, and products can help you keep reimbursement straight.

• Assignment — Agreement in which a service or supply provider accepts the approved Medicare amount of payment as payment in full
• Capitation — Payment method in which an established amount is payable regardless of actual services provided
• CMN (certificate of medical necessity) — Required by Medicare to document the need for medical equipment or supplies
• CMS (Centers for Medicare and Medicaid Services) — Government agency responsible for Medicare and parts of Medicaid; maintains Healthcare Common Procedure Coding System (HCPCS)
• DME (durable medical equipment) — Equipment, such as a walker, cane, or vacuum-assisted therapy device, generally used for a medical purpose
• DMERC (durable medical equipment regional carrier) — Four regional carriers that govern and process Medicare B claims
• DRGs (diagnosis related groups) — Grouping system used by payment sources to classify inpatient hospital services based on a primary diagnosis, secondary diagnoses, demographics, procedures, and possible complications
• HCPCS (Healthcare Common Procedure Coding System) — Coding set used for reimbursement of wound care products
• HHRG (Home Health Resource Groups) — Eighty groups by which home health care patients are classified
• ICD-9 (International Classification of Diseases, Revision 9) — Universal coding system for diagnoses
• OASIS (Outcome and Assessment Information Set) — Required tool used by Medicare-certified home health agencies to identify and document patient data
• Per Diem Reimbursement — reimbursement that's fixed on a set rate per day
• PPS (prospective payment system) — Payment program in which rates are predetermined and providers are reimbursed regardless of the incurred costs
• RUG (resource utilization groups) — Classification system used in nursing facilities to determine a per diem payment rate based on the patient's functional status and acuity
• SNF — skilled nursing facility

Claims for services and products are submitted using a coding system known as the *Healthcare Common Procedure Coding System,* or HCPCS. Current Procedural Terminology codes, which are commonly called CPT codes, are used to bill services. You may encounter several additional reimbursement terms and acronyms. (See *Recognizing reimbursement terms.*)

Medicaid

Medicaid is a medical assistance program for indigent individuals who are elderly, blind, or disabled and for needy families with dependent children. Although conjointly funded through federal and state regulations, it's administered by state agencies. Reimbursement guidelines vary for each state and in each practice setting.

Managed care

Managed care is a health insurance program that combines benefits presented through Medicare and Medicare Plus Choice. Medicare

Plus Choice combines Medicare and private insurance programs—such as health maintenance organizations and preferred provider organizations programs—that may provide benefits not covered by Medicare. Reimbursement is based on fee structures established by each program.

Private pay

Private insurance reimbursement and benefits are also provided in a wide variety of ways. Like the other programs, they have established contracts to pay for services furnished by providers based on reasonable charges. Reasonable charges may include whatever is considered necessary to provide services related to patient care.

Documentation strategies

Health insurance payers are directly involved in treatment decisions because they make decisions regarding payment for medical services and supplies. The fact is, most denials of reimbursement result from insufficient or inconsistent documentation.

Write right

Assessment and documentation are used to determine the patient's care plan and reimbursement decisions. The information used in making care plan and payment decisions comes from the data you provide. Make sure your documentation:
• clearly supports the clinical assessment
• accurately recounts a succession of outcomes related to patient care
• supports payment.

Progress is imperative

Outcome tracking and reevaluation of the care plan are used to track the healing of a patient's wound. They must be done to avoid reimbursement denial. To maximize reimbursement, the practitioner must properly stage and assess wounds and document the patient's progress. Third-party payers no longer pay for continuous wound treatment. They want to see evidence of progress and healing.

Documentation may seem overwhelming but it's incredibly important. Remember, most reimbursement denials result from insufficient or inconsistent documentation.

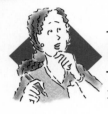

Quick quiz

1. Standards of wound care practice are derived from:
    A.   AHRQ.
    B.   HCPCS.
    C.   Medicare.
    D.   Private insurance companies.

Answer: A. The standards of wound care practice are derived from the AHRQ. The *Patient Care Partnership*, facility- and unit-specific policies and procedures, job descriptions, the AHA's *Standards of Clinical Nursing Practice*, and state nurse practice acts and guidelines also contribute to wound care practice standards.

2. Which agency sponsored the development of *Clinical Practice Guidelines* on the prevention and treatment of pressure ulcers?
    A.   Centers for Disease Control and Prevention
    B.   Agency for Healthcare Research and Quality
    C.   National Institutes of Health
    D.   Food and Drug Administration

Answer: B. The Agency for Healthcare Research and Quality, or AHRQ, is the federal agency for research on major areas of health care. It sponsored the development of the evidence-based *Clinical Practice Guidelines*.

3. Which describes an act of negligence that results in harm?
    A.   Breach of duty
    B.   Proximal cause
    C.   Casual connection
    D.   Established duty

Answer: A. A breach of duty or standard of care must be determined to evaluate whether there has been an act of negligence.

4. The most effective way you can minimize your liability in a malpractice suit is by:
    A.   charting opinions.
    B.   being disrespectful and discourteous.
    C.   charting accurately, clearly, concisely, promptly, and thoroughly.
    D.   being inattentive.

Answer: C. Accurately charting is your best protection to minimize your liability in a malpractice suit.

5. Implementing cost-effective wound care into clinical practice requires knowledge of:
- A. documentation strategies.
- B. *Patient Care Partnership.*
- C. your job description.
- D. HCPCS.

Answer: A. The data you provide guides the care plan and payment decisions.

Scoring

☆☆☆ If you answered all five questions correctly, the ruling is in your favor! You obviously didn't have any issues understanding this chapter.

☆☆ If you answered four questions correctly, don't judge yourself too harshly! But do brush up on the information you missed.

☆ If you answered fewer than four questions correctly, just call this a trial run! Prepare to defend yourself next time by reviewing the chapter.

Appendices and index

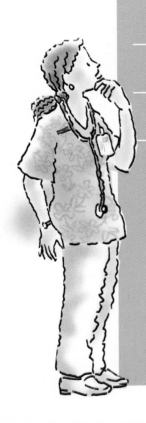

Pressure ulcer prediction and prevention algorithm

This algorithm, developed by the Agency for Healthcare Research and Quality (formerly the Agency for Healthcare Policy and Research), can be used to identify patients at risk for pressure ulcers and to prevent pressure ulcer formation. For detailed guidelines, refer to the *Clinical Practice Guidelines* available online at *www.ahcpr.gov/.*

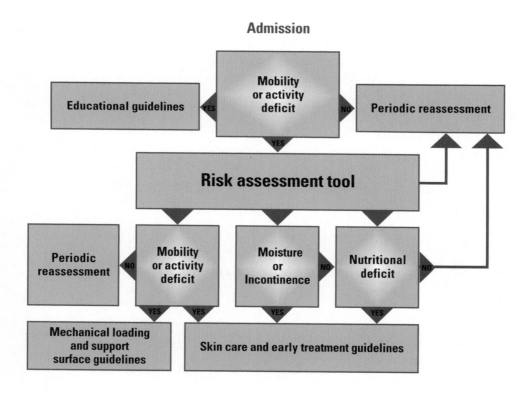

Source: "Pressure Ulcers in Adults: Prediction and Prevention," *Clinical Practice Guideline* Number 3, AHCPR Publication No. 92-0047: May 1992.

Management of pressure ulcers algorithm

This algorithm, developed by the Agency for Healthcare Research and Quality (formerly the Agency for Healthcare Policy and Research), can be used to outline the treatment plan for a patient who has a pressure ulcer. For detailed guidelines, refer to the *Clinical Practice Guidelines* available online at *www.ahcpr.gov/*.

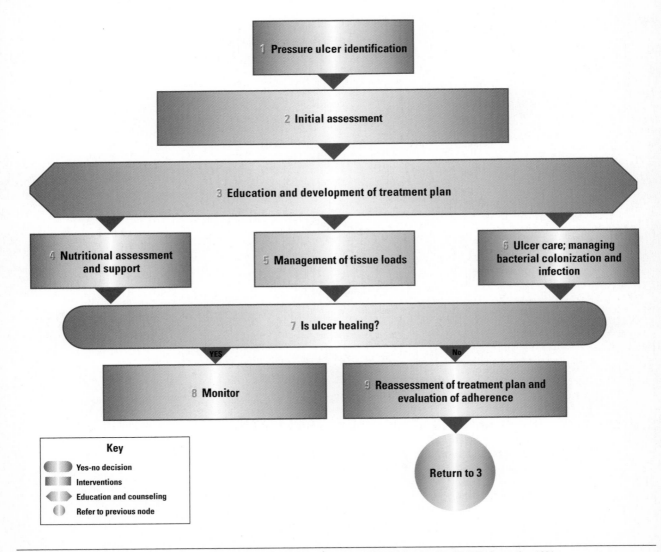

Source: "Treatment of Pressure Ulcers," *Clinical Practice Guideline* Number 15, AHCPR Publication No. 95-0652: December 1994.

Quick guide to wound care dressings

Dressing type	Indications	Products
Alginate	• Wounds with moderate to heavy drainage • Wounds with tunneling	• AlgiCell Calcium Alginate • AlgiDERM Calcium Alginate Dressing or Packing • AlgiSite M • CarboFlex Odor Control Dressing • CarraGinate High G Calcium Alginate Wound Dressing with Acemannan Hydrogel • CarraSorb H Calcium Alginate Wound Dressing • Comfeel SeaSorb • Curasorb • Curasorb Zinc • DermaGinate • Hyperion Advanced Alginate Dressing • KALGINATE Calcium Alginate Wound Dressing • KALTOSTAT Wound Dressing • Maxorb CMC/Alginate Dressing • Melgisorb • Restore CalciCare Wound Care Dressing • Sorbsan Topical Wound Dressing • 3M Tegagen HI and HG Alginate Dressings
Antimicrobial	• Infected wounds	• Acticoat • AcryDerm Silver • Arglaes • Arglaes Powder • AQUACEL AG • Contract • IODOSORB GEL • IODOFLEX • SilverSorb • Silverlon
Biological	• Temporary dressing for skin graft donor sites and burns	• Hyalofill Biopolymeric Wound Dressing • Inerpan Temporary Wound Dressing • Oasis Wound Dressing • Silon Wound Dressing
Collagen	• Chronic, nonhealing, granulated wound beds • Wounds with tunneling	• FIBRACOL PLUS Collagen Wound Dressing with Alginate • Kollagen-Medifil Pads • Kollagen-SkinTemp Sheets

Dressing type	Indications	Products
Composite	• Primary or secondary dressing on wounds with light to moderate drainage • Protection for peripheral and central I.V. lines	• Alldress • CompDress Island Dressing • COVADERM PLUS • DuDress Film Top Island Dressing • MPM Multi-Layered Dressing • Repel Wound Dressing • Stratasorb • TELFA Adhesive Dressing • Telfa Island Dressing • TELFA PLUS Island Dressing • 3M Medipore+Pad Soft Cloth Adhesive Wound Dressing • 3M Tegaderm+Pad Transparent Dressing with Absorbent Pad • Viasorb Wound Dressing
Contact layer	• Wounds with minimal, moderate, and heavy drainage; allows for flow of drainage to a secondary dressing while preventing the dressing from adhering to the wound	• Conformant 2 Wound Veil • DERMANET Wound Contact Layer • Mepitel • N-TERFACE Interpositional Surfacing Material • Profore Wound Contact Layer • Telfa Clear • 3M Tegapore Wound Contact Material • VersaDress Wound Contact Layer
Foam	• Primary or secondary dressing on wounds with minimal to moderate drainage (including around tubes) when a nonadherent surface is important	• Allevyn and Allevyn Adhesive Hydrophilic Polyurethane Foam Dressing • Allevyn Cavity Wound Dressing • Biatain Adhesive Foam Dressing • Biatain Non-Adhesive Foam Dressing • CarraSmart Foam Dressing • Curafoam Plus Foam Dressing • Curafoam Wound Dressing • EPIGARD • Flexzan Topical Wound Dressing • Hydrasorb Foam Wound Dressing • HydroCell Adhesive Foam Dressing • HydroCell Foam Dressing • HydroCell Thin Adhesive Foam Dressing • LO PROFILE FOAM Wound Dressing • Lyofoam A Polyurethane Foam Dressing • Lyofoam C Polyurethane Foam Dressing with Activated Carbon • Lyofoam Extra Polyurethane Foam Dressing • Lyofoam Polyurethane Foam Dressing • Lyofoam T Polyurethane Foam Dressing • Mepilex • Mepilex Border • Mitraflex

Dressing type	Indications	Products
Foam *(continued)*		• Mitraflex Plus • Odor-Absorbent Dressing • Optifoam Adhesive Foam Island Dressing • Optifoam Non-Adhesive Foam Island Dressing • POLYDERM BORDER Hydrophilic Polyurethane Foam Dressing • Polyderm Hydrophilic Polyurethane Foam Dressing • Polyderm Plus Barrier Foam Dressing • PolyMem Adhesive Cloth Dressings • PolyMem Adhesive Film Dressings • PolyMem Calcium Alginate • PolyMem Non-Adhesive Dressings • PolyTube Tube-Site Dressing • PolyWic Cavity Wound Filler • SOF-FOAM Dressing • SorbaCell Foam Dressing • TIELLE Hydropolymer Adhesive Dressing • TIELLE PLUS Hydropolymer Dressing • VigiFOAM Dressing
Hydrocolloid	• Wounds with minimal to moderate drainage, including wounds with necrosis or slough • Secondary dressings (sheet dressings)	• CarraSmart Hydrocolloid with Acemannan Hydrogel • CombiDERM ACD Absorbent Cover Dressing • CombiDERM Non-Adhesive • Comfeel Paste and Powder • Comfeel Plus Contour Dressing • Comfeel Plus Pressure Relief Dressing • Comfeel Plus Triangle Dressing • Comfeel Plus Ulcer Dressing • Comfeel TRIAD Hydrophilic Wound Dressing • DermaFilm HD • DermaFilm Thin • DERMATELL • DERMATELL SECURE • DuoDERM CGF • DuoDERM CGF Border • DuoDERM Extra Thin • DuoDERM Hydroactive Paste • Exuderm • Exuderm LP • Exuderm RCD • Exuderm Sacrum • Exuderm Ultra • Hydrocol • Hydrocol Sacral • Hydrocol Thin • Hyperion Hydrocolloid Dressing

Dressing type	Indications	Products
Hydrocolloid *(continued)*		• MPM Excel Hydrocolloid Wound Dressing • PrimaCol Bordered Hydrocolloid Wound Dressing • PrimaCol Hydrocolloid Dressing • PrimaCol Specialty Hydrocolloid Dressing • PrimaCol Thin Hydrocolloid Dressing • Procol Hydrocolloid Dressing • RepliCare • RepliCare Thin • Restore Cx Wound Care Dressing • Restore Extra Thin Dressing • Restore Plus Wound Care Dressing • Restore Wound Care Dressing • SignaDRESS Hydrocolloid Dressing • Sorbex • Sorbexthin • 3M Tegasorb Hydrocolloid Dressings • 3M Tegasorb THIN Hydrocolloid Dressings • Ulcer Care Dressing • Ultec Hydrocolloid Dressing • Ultec Pro Alginate Hydrocolloid Dressing
Hydrogel	• Dry wounds • Wounds with minimal drainage • Wounds with necrosis	• AcryDerm Moist Hydrophilic Wound Dressing • Amerigel Ointment • Aquaflo • AquaGauze Hydrogel Impregnated Gauze Dressing • Aquasite Amorphous Hydrogel • Aquasite Impregnated Gauze Hydrogel • Aquasite Impregnated Non-Woven Hydrogel • Aquasite Sheet Hydrogel • Aquasorb Hydrogel Wound Dressing • Bandage Roll with ClearSite • Biolex Wound Gel • CarraDres Clear Hydrogel Sheet • CarraGauze Pads and Strips with Acemannan Hydrogel • CarraSmart Gel Wound Dressing with Acemannan Hydrogel • Carrasyn Gel Wound Dressing with Acemannan Hydrogel • Carrasyn Spray Gel Wound Dressing with Acemannan Hydrogel • Carrasyn V with Acemannan Hydrogel • Comfort-Aid • Curafil Gel Wound Dressing and Impregnated Strips • Curagel • CURASOL Gel Wound Dressing • DermaGel Hydrogel Sheet • Dermagran Hydrophilic Wound Dressing • Dermagran Zinc-Saline Hydrogel

Dressing type	Indications	Products
Hydrogel (continued)		• DermaSyn • DiaB Gel with Acemannan Hydrogel • Elasto-Gel • Elasto-Gel Plus • Elta Hydrogel Impregnated Gauze • Elta Hydrovase Wound Gel • Elta Wound Gel • FlexiGel • Gentell Hydrogel • Hypergel • Hyperion Hydrogel Gauze Dressing • Hyperion Hydrophilic Wound Dressing • Hyperion Hydrophilic Wound Gel • Iamin Hydrating Gel • IntraSite Gel • MPM Excel Gel • MPM GelPad Hydrogel Saturated Dressing • MPM Regenecare • Normlgel • NU-GEL Collagen Wound Gel • PanoGauze Hydrogel Impregnated Gauze Dressing • PanoPlex Hydrogel Wound Dressing • Phyto Derma Wound Gel • Purilon Gel • RadiaDres Gel Sheet with Acemannan Hydrogel • RadiaGel with Acemannan Hydrogel • Restore Hydrogel Dressing • SAF-Gel Hydrating Dermal Wound Dressing • Skintegrity Amorphous Hydrogel • Skintegrity Hydrogel Impregnated Gauze • SoloSite Gel Conformable Wound Dressing • SoloSite Wound Gel • TenderWet Gel Pad • 3M Tegagel Hydrogel Wound Fillers • TOE-AID Toe and Nail Dressing • Ultrex Gel Wound Dressing • Vigilon Primary Wound Dressing • Wound Dressing with ClearSite • WOUN'DRES Collagen Hydrogel
Specialty absorptive	• Infected or noninfected wounds with heavy drainage	• AQUACEL • BAND-AID Brand Island Surgical Dressings • BreakAway Wound Dressing • CombiDERM ACD Absorbent Cover Dressing • CombiDERM Non-Adhesive • Covaderm Adhesive Wound Dressing

Dressing type	Indications	Products
Specialty absorptive *(continued)*		• CURITY Abdominal Pads • DuPad Abdominal Pads, Open End • DuPad Abdominal Pads, Sealed End • EXU-DRY • Mepore • Multipad Non-Adherent Wound Dressing • Primapore Specialty Absorptive Dressing • Sofsorb Wound Dressing • SURGI-PAD Combine Dressing • TENDERSORB WET-PRUF Abdominal Pads
Transparent film	• Partial-thickness wounds with minimal exudate • Wounds with eschar	• BIOCLUSIVE Select Transparent Dressing • BIOCLUSIVE Transparent Dressing • Blisterfilm • CarraFilm Transparent Film Dressing • CarraSmart Film Transparent Film Dressing • ClearCell Transparent Film Dressing • ClearSite Transparent Membrane • DERMAVIEW • Mefilm • OpSite • OpSite FLEXIGRID • OpSite PLUS • OpSite Post-Op • Polyskin II Transparent Dressing • Polyskin MR Moisture Responsive Transparent Dressing • ProCyte Transparent Film Dressing • Suresite • 3M Tegaderm HP Transparent Dressing • Transeal Transparent Wound Dressing • UniFlex
Wound filler	• Primary dressing on an infected or a noninfected wound with minimal to moderate drainage that requires packing	• AcryDerm STRANDS Absorbent Wound Filler • Bard Absorption Dressing • CarraSorb M Freeze Dried Gel Wound Dressing with Acemannan Hydrogel • Catrix 5 Rejuvenation Cream • Catrix 10 Ointment • Catrix Wound Dressing • FlexiGel Strands Absorbent Wound Dressing • hyCURE • hyCURE SMART GEL • IODOFLEX PAD • IODOSORB GEL • Kollagen-Medifil II Gel • Kollagen-Medifil II Particles • Multidex Maltodextrin Wound Dressing Gel or Powder

Wound and skin assessment tool

When performing a thorough wound and skin assessment, a pictorial demonstration is often helpful to identify the wound site or sites. Using the wound and skin assessment tool here, the practitioner identified that the posterior of the patient's right elbow has a full-thickness pressure ulcer that's red in color.

PATIENT'S NAME (LAST, MIDDLE, FIRST)	ATTENDING PHYSICIAN	ROOM NUMBER	ID NUMBER
Jacobs, Elijah	Dr. A. Nichols	123-4	04113

WOUND ASSESSMENT:

NUMBER	1	2	3	4	5	6
DATE	4/11/07					
TIME	0800					
LOCATION	®️ elbow					
STAGE	III					
APPEARANCE	IN					
SIZE-LENGTH	0.5 cm					
SIZE-WIDTH	1 cm					
COLOR/FLR.	RD					
DRAINAGE	0					
ODOR	0					
VOLUME	0					
INFLAMMATION	0					
SIZE INFLAM.						

KEY

Stage:
- I. Red or discolored
- II. Skin break/blister
- III. Sub 'Q' tissue
- IV. Muscle and/or bone

Appearance:
- D = Depth
- E = Eschar
- G = Granulation
- IN = Inflammation
- NEC = Necrotic
- PK = Pink
- SL = Slough
- TN = Tunneling
- UND = Undermining
- MX = Mixed (specify)

Color of Wound

Floor:
- RD = Red
- Y = Yellow
- BLK = Black
- MX = Mixed (specify)

Drainage:
- 0 = None
- SR = Serous
- SS = Serosanguineous
- BL = Blood
- PR = Purulent

Odor:
- 0 = None
- MLD = Mild
- FL = Foul

Volume:
- 0 = None
- SC = Scant
- MOD = Moderate
- LG = Large

Inflammation:
- 0 = None
- PK = Pink
- RD = Red

258

WOUND ANATOMICAL LOCATION:

(circle affected area)

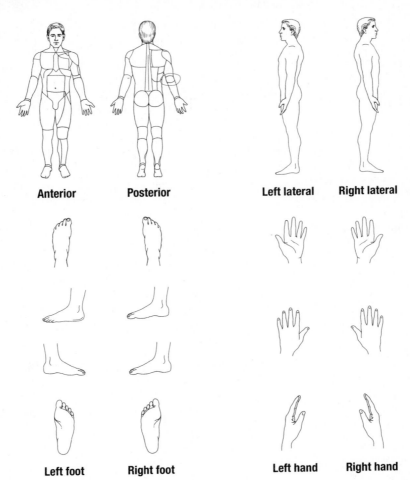

| Anterior | Posterior | | Left lateral | Right lateral |

| Left foot | Right foot | | Left hand | Right hand |

Wound care protocol: _Clean wound with NSS._

Signature: _Andrea Smith, RN_   Date _4/11/07_

Glossary

abrasion
a wearing away of the skin through some mechanical process, such as friction or trauma

abscess
a circumscribed collection of pus that forms in tissue as a result of acute or chronic localized infection and is associated with tissue destruction and, in many cases, swelling

acute wound
any wound that's new or progressing as expected

albumin
a large protein molecule that's water-soluble and provides colloid osmotic pressure

alginate
a nonwoven, highly absorptive dressing that's manufactured from seaweed (kelp)

angiogenesis
the formation and regeneration of blood vessels

antimicrobial
an agent that kills microbes or inhibits their growth

autolysis
the breakdown of tissues or cells by the body's own mechanisms, such as enzymes or white blood cells

bacteria
one-celled microorganisms that break down dead tissue, have no true nucleus, and reproduce by cell division

blanchable erythema
a reddened area of the skin that temporarily turns white or pale when pressure is applied with a fingertip; also known as reactive hyperemia

bottoming out
flattening of the support surface of the body, determined by the caregiver placing an outstretched hand (palm up) under the mattress overlay, below the part of the body at risk for ulcer formation (If the caregiver feels that the support material is less than 1-inch thick at this site, the patient has "bottomed out.")

burn
an acute wound that's caused by exposure to thermal extremes, caustic chemicals, electricity, or radiation

cellulitis
cellular or connective tissue inflammation that's characterized by redness, swelling, and tenderness

chemical debridement
the topical application of biological enzymes to break down devitalized tissue

chronic wound
any wound that isn't healing in a timely fashion (healing has slowed or stopped)

collagen
the main supportive protein of skin, tendon, bone, cartilage, and connective tissue

colloid osmotic pressure
the force that prevents fluid from leaking out of blood vessels into nearby tissues

colonized
contaminated with bacteria

contamination
the presence of bacteria, microorganisms, or other foreign material in or on tissues (wounds with bacterial counts of 10 or fewer organisms per gram of tissue are usually considered contaminated; those with higher counts are generally considered infected)

cytotoxic agents
compounds that destroy both diseased and healthy cells, which may be used to clean wounds; examples include povidone-iodine, Dakin's solution, and hydrogen peroxide

dead space
an area of tissue destruction or loss that extends out from the main body of the wound, leaving a cavity or tract (this area is lightly packed to avoid superficial closure that can lead to abscess formation)

debridement
the removal of necrotic (dead) tissue to allow underlying healthy tissue to regenerate

debris
the remains of broken down or damaged cells or tissue

dehiscence
a partial or total separation of skin and tissue layers

demyelination
the destruction of a nerve's myelin sheath, which interferes with normal nerve conduction

dermis
the thick, inner layer of skin

diabetes mellitus
a metabolic disorder characterized by hyperglycemia resulting from lack of insulin, lack of insulin effect, or both

differentiation
the remodeling of collagen from a gel-like consistency to a mature scar (this maturation imparts mechanical strength to the tissue)

drainage
the fluid produced by a wound, which may contain serum, cellular debris, bacteria, leukocytes, pus, or blood

enzyme
a protein that acts as a catalyst to induce chemical changes in other substances

epidermis
the outermost layer of the skin

epithelialization
the regeneration of epidermis across the wound surface

erythema
an inflammatory redness of the skin caused by engorged capillaries

eschar
nonviable (dead) wound tissue that's characterized by a dry, leathery, black crust

evisceration
the abrupt protrusion of underlying visceral organs from a wound

excoriation
abrasions or scratches on the skin

exudate
any fluid that has been extruded from tissue or capillaries, usually due to injury or inflammation; it's characteristically high in protein and white blood cells

fascia
a band of white fibrous tissue that lies deep in relation to the skin and forms a supportive sheath for muscles and various body organs

fibrin
an insoluble protein, formed from fibrinogen by the proteolytic action of thrombin, that's essential in blood clotting

fibroblasts
the most common cells in connective tissue; responsible for making fibers and extracellular matrix, which provides support to cells

fistula
an abnormal passage between two organs or between an organ and the skin

foam
a spongelike polymer dressing with some absorptive properties that may be adherent or impregnated or coated with other materials

friction
the act of rubbing one surface against another; may lead to the physiologic wearing away of tissue

full-thickness wound
any wound that penetrates completely through the skin into underlying tissues; adipose tissue, muscle, tendon, or bone may be exposed

gauze
a woven cotton or synthetic fabric dressing that's absorptive and permeable to water, water vapor, and oxygen and may be impregnated with petroleum, antiseptics, or other agents

granulation
the formation of soft, pink, fleshy projections during the healing process in a wound not healing by primary intention, consisting of new capillaries surrounded by fibrous collagen; tissue appears reddened from the rich blood supply

healing ridge
a buildup of collagen fibers that begins to form during the inflammatory phase of wound healing and peaks during the proliferation phase

hemorrhage
bleeding (may be internal or external)

hydrocolloid
an adhesive, moldable wafer dressing that's made of carbohydrates, has a nonpermeable waterproof backing, and may have some absorptive properties

hydrogel
a water-based nonadherent dressing that has some absorptive qualities

hydrophilic
the ability to readily absorb moisture

hypoxia
the reduction of oxygen in body tissues to below normal levels

induration
tissue firmness that may occur around a wound margin following blanchable erythema or chronic venous congestion

infection

a pathogenic contamination that's reacted against but can't be controlled by the body's immune system

inflammation

a localized protective response elicited by injury or destruction of tissue that's characterized by heat, redness, swelling, pain, and loss of function

insulin

a hormone secreted into the blood by the islets of Langerhans in the pancreas that promotes the storage of glucose, among other functions

irrigation

cleaning tissue and removing cell debris and drainage from an open wound by flushing it with a stream of liquid

ischemia

deficient blood supply to a body organ or tissue

lymphedema

the chronic swelling of a body part from accumulation of interstitial fluid secondary to obstruction of lymphatic vessels or lymph nodes

maceration

the softening of a solid as it's soaked in fluid (in wounds, maceration is indicated by whitened tissue)

macrophage

a highly phagocytic cell that's stimulated by inflammation

mechanical debridement

the removal of foreign material and devitalized or contaminated tissue from a wound by physical force rather than by chemical (enzymatic) or natural (autolytic) forces; examples include wet-to-dry dressings, pulsatile lavage, and whirlpool therapy

melanin

a dark skin pigment that filters ultraviolet radiation and is produced and dispersed by specialized cells called *melanocytes*

myelin

a lipidlike substance that surrounds the axon of myelinated nerve fibers and permits normal neurologic conduction

necrosis

cell or tissue death

neuron

a highly specialized conductor cell that receives and transmits electrochemical nerve impulses

neutrophil

a type of white blood cell that's responsible for phagocytosis

nonblanching erythema

a redness of the skin that persists when gentle pressure is applied to it and released

nutritional assessment

an assessment of the relationship between nutrients consumed and energy expended, especially when illness or surgery compromises a patient's intake or alters his metabolic requirements (includes a dietary history, physical assessment, anthropometric measurements, and diagnostic tests)

partial-thickness wound

any wound that involves only the epidermal layer of the skin or extends through the epidermis and into — but not through — the dermis

pathogen

any microorganism capable of producing disease

peripheral vascular disease

a group of disorders that affect the blood vessels outside the heart or the lymphatic vessels

phagocyte

a cell that ingests microorganisms, other cells, and foreign particles

phagocytosis

the engulfment of microorganisms, other cells, and foreign particles by a phagocyte

polyneuropathy

damage to multiple types of nerves

pressure

a force that's applied vertically or perpendicular to a surface

pressure gradient

the difference in pressure between two points (the transmission of pressure from one tissue to another causes an increase in pressure to those tissues that are deepest)

pressure ulcers

wounds that are the clinical manifestation of localized tissue death due to lack of blood flow in areas under pressure

primary dressing

a dressing that's placed directly on the wound bed

protein
a large, complex molecule composed of amino acids, which are essential for tissue growth and repair

pus
a thick, yellowish fluid that's composed of albuminous substances, thin fluid, and leukocytes

reactive hyperemia
an increased amount of blood in a body part following stoppage and subsequent restoration of the blood supply

sebaceous gland
a saclike structure that produces sebum

sebum
a fatty substance that lubricates and softens the skin

sharp debridement
the removal of foreign material or devitalized (dead) tissue using a sharp instrument such as a scalpel

shearing force
a mechanical force that runs parallel, rather than perpendicular, to an area of skin (deep tissues feel the brunt of this force)

sinus tract
a cavity or channel that permits the drainage of wound contents

skin sealant
a clear liquid that creates a film barrier to seal and protect the skin from trauma

slough
nonviable tissue that's loosely attached; characterized by stringlike, moist, necrotic debris; and yellow, green, or gray in color

subcutaneous tissue
a layer of loose connective tissue below the epidermis and dermis that contains major blood vessels, lymph vessels, and nerves; also known as the *hypodermis*

surgical wound
a healthy and uncomplicated break in the skin's continuity resulting from surgery

tendon
a fibrous cord of connective tissue that attaches the muscle to bone or cartilage and enables bones to move when skeletal muscles contract

tensile strength
the maximum force or pressure that can be applied to a wound without causing it to break apart

tissue
a large group of individual cells that perform a certain function

tissue biopsy
the use of a sharp instrument to obtain a sample of skin, muscle, or bone for diagnostic purposes

transparent film
a clear, adherent, nonabsorptive dressing that's permeable to oxygen and water vapor

traumatic wound
a sudden, unplanned injury to the skin that can range from minor to severe

tunnel
an extension of the wound bed into adjacent tissue; also known as a *sinus tract*

undermining
a tunneling effect or pocket under the edges of a wound that's caused by the pressure gradient transmitted from the body surface to the bone

vascular wound
any chronic wound that stems from peripheral vascular disease in the venous, arterial, or lymphatic system

wet-to-dry dressing
a dressing that's used in debridement; gauze moistened with normal saline solution is applied to the wound and then removed once the gauze becomes dry and adheres to the wound bed

wound
any break in the skin

Selected references

Ayello, E.A., et al. "Nursing 2005 Wound Care Survey Report," *Nursing2005* 35(6):36-45, June 2005.

Bechara, F.G., et al. "Shave Therapy for Chronic Venous Ulcers: A Guideline for Surgical Management and Postoperative Wound Care," *Plastic Surgical Nursing* 26(1):29-34, January-March 2006.

Brown, P., and Maloy, J.P. *Quick Reference to Wound Care*, 2nd ed. Sudbury, Mass.: Jones & Bartlett Publishers, Inc., 2005.

Cutting, K.F., and White, R.J. "Criteria for Identifying Wound Infection Revisited," *Ostomy/Wound Management* 51(1): 28-34, January 2005.

Hess, C.T. *Clinical Guide to Wound Care*, 5th ed. Philadelphia: Lippincott Williams & Wilkins, 2005.

Hess, C.T. "The Art of Skin and Wound Care Documentation," *Advances in Skin & Wound Care* 18(1):43-53, January-February 2005.

Marston, W.A. "Risk Factors Associated with Healing Chronic Diabetic Foot Ulcers: The Importance of Hyperglycemia," *Ostomy/Wound Management* 52(3):26-39, March 2006.

Maylor, M.E. "Establishing Nurses' Preferences in Wound Assessment: A Concept Evaluation," *Journal of Clinical Nursing* 15(4):444-50, April 2006.

McIntosh, C.D., and Thomson, C.E. "Honey Dressing Versus Paraffin Tulle Gras Following Toenail Surgery," *Journal of Wound Care* 15(3):133-36, March 2006.

Mendez-Eastman, S. "Use Negative-Pressure Wound Therapy for Positive Results," *Nursing2005* 35(5):48-50, May 2005.

Molan, P.C. "The Evidence Supporting the Use of Honey as a Wound Dressing," *International Journal of Lower Extremity Wounds* 5(1):40-54, March 2006.

Phelps, J.R., et al. "A Case Study of Negative-Pressure Wound Therapy to Manage Acute Necrotizing Fasciitis," *Ostomy/Wound Management* 52(3):54-59, March 2006.

Pieper, B. "Wound Management in Vulnerable Populations," *Rehabilitation Nursing* 30(3): 100-105, May-June 2005.

Posthauer, M.E. "Hydration: Does It Play a Role in Wound Healing?" *Advances in Skin & Wound Care* 19(2):97-102, March 2006.

Salcido, R.S. "Using Our Senses in Wound Care," *Advances in Skin & Wound Care* 18(1):8-11, January-February 2005.

Sargent, R.L. "Management of Blisters in the Partial-Thickness Burn: An Integrative Research Review" *Journal of Burn Care and Research* 27(1):66-81, January-February 2006.

Schuster, R., et al. "The Use of Vacuum-Assisted Closure Therapy for the Treatment of a Large Infected Facial Wound," *The American Surgeon* 72(2):129-31, February 2006.

Smith, S. "Successful Outcomes With the H.E.A.L. Program," *Ostomy/Wound Management* 52(3):40-53, March 2006.

Sweitzer, S.M., et al. "What Is the Future of Diabetic Wound Care?" *The Diabetes Educator* 32(2):197-210, March-April 2006.

Vlahakis, N.E. "Is Erythropoietin the Key to Optimize Wound Healing?" *Critical Care Medicine* 34(4):1279-80, April 2006.

Index

i refers to an illustration; t refers to a table; bold numbers refer to color pages.

i refers to an illustration; t refers to a table; bold numbers refer to color pages.

i refers to an illustration; t refers to a table; bold numbers refer to color pages.

i refers to an illustration; t refers to a table; bold numbers refer to color pages.

i refers to an illustration; t refers to a table; bold numbers refer to color pages.

i refers to an illustration; t refers to a table; bold numbers refer to color pages.

Notes

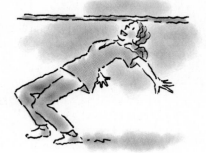

Notes

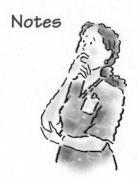